Easy Interpretation of Biostatistics

Easy Interpretation of Biostatistics

The Vital Link to Applying Evidence in Medical Decisions

Gail F. Dawson, MD, MS, FAAEP
University of Michigan, Ann Arbor MI
Wayne State University, Detroit MI

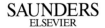

SAUNDERS
ELSEVIER

1600 John F. Kennedy Blvd.
Ste 1800
Philadelphia, PA 19103-2899

EASY INTERPRETATION OF BIOSTATISTICS:
The Vital Link to Applying Evidence in Medical Decisions   ISBN: 978-1-4160-3142-0
Copyright © 2008 by Saunders, an imprint of Elsevier Inc.

Notice

Knowledge and best practice in this field are constantly changing. As new research and experience broaden our knowledge, changes in practice, treatment and drug therapy may become necessary or appropriate. Readers are advised to check the most current information provided (i) on procedures featured or (ii) by the manufacturer of each product to be administered, to verify the recommended dose or formula, the method and duration of administration, and contraindications. It is the responsibility of the practitioner, relying on their own experience and knowledge of the patient, to make diagnoses, to determine dosages and the best treatment for each individual patient, and to take all appropriate safety precautions. To the fullest extent of the law, neither the Publisher nor the Author assumes any liability for any injury and/or damage to persons or property arising out of or related to any use of the material contained in this book.

The Publisher

Library of Congress Cataloging-in-Publication Data
Dawson, Gail F.
   Easy interpretation of biostatistics: the vital link to applying evidence in medical decisions / Gail F. Dawson.—1st ed.
      p.; cm.
   Includes bibliographical references and index.
   ISBN 978-1-4160-3142-0
1. Medicine—Research—Statistical methods. 2. Biometry. I. Title.
   [DNLM: 1. Biometry—methods. 2. Data Interpretation, Statistical. 3. Epidemiologic Methods. WA 950 D2725e 2008]
R853.S7D39 2008
610.72'7—dc22   2007000829

Acquisitions Editor: James Merritt
Developmental Editor: Nicole DiCicco
Project Manager: Bryan Hayward
Design Direction: Gene Harris

Working together to grow
libraries in developing countries

www.elsevier.com | www.bookaid.org | www.sabre.org

ELSEVIER   BOOK AID International   Sabre Foundation

Printed in the United States of America
Last digit is the print number: 9 8 7 6 5 4 3 2 1

This book is dedicated to all those who like to teach,
for the sheer joy that comes from sharing the knowledge.

A special thanks to the people in my life
who have touched me with their wisdom,
dedication, laughter, and compassion, and especially to...

Alan, Gary, Diane,
Dennis, and Joyce
Drew, Alex, Carl,
and Jim

for their love and support.

Our life is frittered away with detail ... Simplify. Simplify.
—Henry David Thoreau

PREFACE

We are fortunate to live in an era where incredible advances in science and technology have made it possible to extend human lives longer than ever before. The appropriate use of these tools has had an astounding impact on the human condition. Because of proper health care, life expectancies have almost doubled in the last century. In addition to living longer, people are also more productive in their later years due to their overall better health.

Health care workers provide the means by which these advances can be applied to the population. Through research, individualized patient care, and health care policy we attempt to provide the best care for the largest number of people. Quite simply, there are only two reasons why we, as health care professionals, do what we do: We help people *live longer*, and we help people *feel better*. Any intervention we recommend or perform, from the simple daily aspirin to the complex stem cell transplant, should be justified by contributing to at least one of these two categories. This is the common mission of health care providers.

When we recommend an intervention, we do it with the intention of a good outcome for a particular individual. That is to say, we want the individual to live longer, or feel better, or both. However, a certain proportion of individuals will have complications as a result of the intervention, even when screening is done to exclude those who are likely to have an adverse outcome. Does this mean the intervention should be abandoned? Not if we can show that the majority of those undergoing the intervention will have an improvement in their condition that is worth the risk of the adverse events that might occur. In this way, the live longer/feel better requirement is fulfilled because the benefit to the larger population takes precedence over the adverse events of the few.

My son Alex and I were recently musing on the great inventions of the last few centuries. He thought the automobile was a major contributor, since it provided a huge opportunity for a better life for many people. Because of mass employment in the factories, there was a shift in the population to the cities where common resources such as water, sewers, and power could be concentrated. The workers enjoyed steady substantial wages and could afford more amenities. The limited workday allowed more time for entertainment for the employees. In their free time, they were able to socialize more often by taking advantage of the transportation available. The auto industry was also indirectly responsible for high quality, consistent health care through the bargaining power of its unions. I had to agree with Alex. It is undeniably true that the automobile had (and still does have) a huge impact on the quality of life for many people.

There are many other inventions that have contributed to the benefit of humankind. I'm sure you can name a few. My own personal favorite is the remote control. (There is a gleeful delight in making something happen without getting up. You don't even have to ask nicely!) In the global context, however, I hold the most respect for this invention: *The development of the science of biostatistics and its application to medicine.*

Biostatistics allows us to quantify live longer/feel better. This is the way we confirm that the interventions we recommend, which consume our precious time, energy, and resources, are truly the best course for the most people. By measuring outcomes using mathematical values, we can weigh the advantage of one intervention over another, or compare an intervention to not doing anything. The end result is our verification for why we do what we do. It simply benefits the most people. The application of this science is reflected in the increased lifespan and ample quality of life that we currently enjoy.

As you can see, the benefits of this applied science are not to be underestimated. Biostatistics provides the framework for all types of medical research, and allows us to convert this knowledge into practices that contribute to the betterment of the human race. This has resulted in an enormous improvement on our ability to live longer and feel better. On a philosophical level, however, applied biostatistics has an even more noble justification.

There are currently several theories on how to assess intelligence. There is some disagreement on the exact definition of the word intelligence, especially from different sides of the globe. Eastern cultures tend to emphasize self-knowledge and interpersonal relationships, while the Western notion centers on learning skills.[1] Despite these differences in philosophical beliefs, however, there is a general consensus that intelligence involves more than just memorizing and repeating information, like an animal performing circus tricks. It's commonly accepted that intelligence includes the ability to reason and make judgements. The more intelligent beings not only assimilate information, but also process it and use it to their advantage. Some psychologists measure intelligence by a creature's ability to communicate, such as a pack of wolves might do while hunting prey. Others maintain it is a marker of how well animals use tools to manipulate the environment to their benefit, like a sea otter using a rock to crack open a clam to eat the morsel inside.

Another proposed manifestation of intelligence is the ability to process information, both past and present, to determine a course of action that is least likely to result in death or injury (recognize the live longer/feel better theme?). This theory states that the most intelligent species are those who recognize and utilize the fact that they can affect their own outcome by altering how they react in a given situation. When they encounter a new situation, they analyze the circumstances and integrate information that was learned in the past to decide on the best course of action. Biostatistics allows us to collect and logically utilize data to increase our knowledge of a given situation, so we can apply it in a manner that will provide the greatest benefit. It is a valid argument, then, that the application of biostatistics is the quintessential measure of intelligence. It provides the paradigm within which we, the human race, can achieve our utmost intellectual potential.

Biostatistics is a stalwart science built on a framework of logic and reason. It justifies the decisions we make for our patients. It guides us in our journey as we strive toward fairness in the development of health care policy. As we have seen, it also invites some very intriguing philosophical ideas. I hope I have instilled some of the enthusiasm that I hold for this discipline. It's very cool stuff. Let's go!

Gail F. Dawson

---

1. Sternberg R. J. and Kaufman J. C. 1998. Human Abilities. *Annu. Rev. Psychol.* 49:479–502

CONTENTS

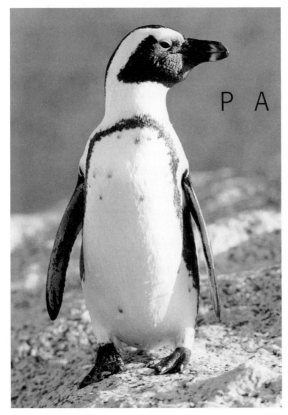

Learning the Basics

Strange how much you've got to know
before you know how little you know.
—*Anonymous*

INTRODUCTION TO PART I

As professionals in the field of health care, it is important to understand why we do what we do. Patients look to us to provide them with the scenario for the best possible outcome. The science of biostatistics is used to verify the approach that we recommend to individuals, based on studies done on larger populations of people who have similar characteristics.

The prototypical application of biostatistics is the clinical trial. Subjects are divided into two or more groups, each group undergoing a different treatment. We quantify the response to a given treatment. Mathematical formulas are then used to compare the degree of difference between the groups. If we can demonstrate a significant difference, we know which pathway is more likely to result in a favorable outcome, and we can then make a recommendation guided by these results.

Health care providers often rely on scientific studies to furnish answers to the question, "What should I tell this patient to do?" In order to accurately counsel a patient and recommend treatment, it is essential to know how to use the results of studies that have been published in journals. This wealth of information is referred to as "evidence." In general, it is more reliable than operating on your own or your colleagues' personal experience.

Biostatistics is also used in determining health policy. Administrators rely on studies to guide them in developing programs designed to provide the most effective care at the lowest cost. For instance, screening programs should be able to demonstrate a significant advantage before they are put into effect. Insurance companies use this information to assure that they are distributing the finances in a way that benefits the most people.

This science has also found its way into the courtroom. Judges are being pressured to admit only the soundest evidence pertaining to the facts in a trial involving medical issues, rather than relying on who can tell the most convincing story or give the most flamboyant performance. A recent Supreme Court ruling[1] determined that federal trial judges who preside over questions of litigation now have a "gate keeping" responsibility to scrutinize expert testimony for evidential reliability and scientific validity. In order to evaluate the admissibility of proffered expert testimony, it's necessary to have a working knowledge of the simple concepts of biostatistics which are used to interpret data and validate decisions.

Journalists who report on medically related issues need to understand these concepts as well, since readers depend on the press to provide reliable information. A responsible reporter should be able to present the public with an accurate interpretation of a scientific study. Invalid conclusions and scare tactics only confuse and alienate an already wary audience. In fact, it behooves all of us who read the press to be able to critique the logic that was used in an article, and to decide independently if the data support the conclusion of the investigators.

The published medical literature provides a wealth of information to help guide our decisions in all of these arenas. However, many of us have had inadequate training when it comes to interpreting the literature. We feel intimidated by the intricate statistical formulas that are used. We are uncomfortable with terms like "confidence interval" and "power" since they are based on concepts that seem quite complex. Since few of us have had extensive training in statistics, it can be confusing to interpret the medical literature.

Imagine yourself in an unfamiliar city, trying to get from one place to another. Instead of randomly setting out, you find it's much more effective to obtain a map of the city to help you navigate. As long as you know how to interpret the map, you can use it to your benefit. You did not create the map. You left that to the cartographer, and trusted that s/he recorded the information accurately. However, you have the necessary skills to interpret the map so you can reach your destination.

Understanding the concepts of biostatistics is like possessing the knowledge that allows you to read a map correctly. The skills you need to interpret the literature will let you get the answer you seek to guide you in your decisions and recommendations. It is not necessary to know the mathematics behind the statistical test. You leave that to the statistical experts. You trust them to provide you with the most appropriate test for the type of data and with reliable test results. Not all health care professionals can be statisticians, nor do they need to be. With a basic understanding of the concepts that are employed, you should be able to navigate easily through the medical literature.

The purpose of this book is to present the concepts of biostatistics in a simple, organized fashion that is easy to understand. Each chapter focuses on a single concept, and the information is assimilated in a stepwise fashion so it is reinforced as you proceed. The principal concepts are emphasized, while the mathematical formulas have been kept to a minimum. This is not a textbook of statistics. (That wouldn't be nearly as much fun!) The purpose is not to transform you into a biostatistician, but rather to provide you with the skills necessary to confidently interpret the literature so you may practice evidence-based medicine or apply the skills to a related profession. You will learn the logic behind the process of inference and develop a working vocabulary that will allow you to participate in discussions regarding the medical literature. You'll also pick up a few historical anecdotes along the way.

This book is produced with you in mind. I am aware that many of you have time constraints, so the chapters are concise and focus on the major concepts. I also realize that many health care professionals practice in an environment that allows a few minutes of potentially reflective time between scheduled events such as rounds, lectures, procedures, or meetings. This book is purposely designed so these brief time intervals can be used effectively by reviewing the key points.

The chapters are built on concepts. Graphs have been used whenever possible to illustrate ideas. It's recommended that you understand one chapter thoroughly before moving on to the next. At the end of each chapter are several review questions that focus on the key points. Cover the answer and try to come up with the best response. This method reinforces the learning process. If you need to look back through the text, then feel free to do so. You will understand the material better if you attempt a response before looking at the answer provided. Some questions may have more than one correct response, but the answers should be interchangeable. Let's try a few right now.

REVIEW QUESTIONS

1. We use biostatistics to justify _____.

   why we do what we do
   what we recommend to
   patients

2. All types of _____ use biostatistics to make treatment or policy decisions.

   people, professionals,
   practitioners

3. Biostatistics uses mathematical formulas to _____ in different treatment groups in the same population.

compare outcomes or responses or degree of differences

4. In general, treatment or policy decisions based on _____ is more reliable than personal experience.

evidence

5. It is not necessary to know the _____ in order to understand simple concepts of biostatistics.

mathematical formulas

6. I like understanding the concepts of biostatistics because _____.

it's fun
it's intriguing
it helps me advise my patients
it guides me in health care decisions
it helps me determine the reliability of what I read in press
it allows me to judge the strength of the evidence

REFERENCE

1. Daubert v. Merrell Dow Pharmaceuticals 509 US 579 [1993].

CHAPTER 1

Measures of Disease

The premise underlying Epidemiology is that disease, illness, and ill health are not randomly distributed in a population.

—*Leon Gordis*[1]

The early disciples of medicine were fascinated by the observation that certain types of diseases tend to cluster. They searched for explanations to account for the trends they saw. They felt that if they could understand the process of the spread of disease, then perhaps illness could be prevented by avoiding the precipitating factors.

To have a successful prevention or treatment program, however, it was necessary to have a way to measure rates of disease. Only then would it be possible to verify that an intervention had a beneficial effect on the transmission of disease. The science of epidemiology evolved from the study of disease patterns and the desire to control disease rates. It uses biostatistical methods to study trends in large populations and to evaluate the effectiveness of treatment and prevention programs. It is helpful to know the basic methods of disease measurement to get an appreciation for the burden of disease on a population and to understand how biostatistics is applied to this science.

Epidemiology is the study of the distribution of illness in populations, based on the fact that diseases often present in a certain focus of people. This is especially apparent with infectious diseases that are transmitted from person to person, such as tuberculosis. The tendency for diseases to be seen in certain populations is not necessarily based on location, however. Clustering may also depend on other environmental factors, which are referred to as exposures. For instance, smokers tend to get certain lung diseases that non-smokers do not, no matter where they live. Epidemiology attempts to identify the exposures that are associated with disease and to control these factors, thereby reducing the disease rates. Through surveillance methods we can also identify potential epidemics, especially in reportable diseases.

INCIDENCE AND PREVALENCE

Diseases can be measured by quantifying the incidence rates at which they occur. The word *rate* implies that something is happening over time. Incidence is defined as the number of *new* cases of a disease that occur over a certain period of time, usually

1 year, divided by the number of people at risk. For example, if 15 people develop influenza out of 100 who are exposed over a year, the incidence of new cases of influenza is 0.15/year. Because incidence measures the occurrence of an event (disease) over time, it is a measurement of the *risk* of getting the disease if you belong to the population.

- *Incidence is the number of new cases of a disease divided by the number of people at risk for the disease, over a given period of time.*
- *Incidence is a measure of risk.*

Incidence is used to track the baseline rates of disease and to measure the effectiveness of prevention programs such as immunizations. *Hemophilus influenzae* is a bacterium that can cause meningitis and epiglottis in young children. These are both potentially life-threatening illnesses. When the *Hemophilus influenzae* vaccination was introduced, the incidence of these diseases was markedly decreased (Figure 1-1). In addition to an overall decline in incidence, a shift was observed in the average age of presentation of these diseases—from very young children who were now protected by the vaccination, to older children who had not been immunized (Figure 1-2). If the incidence of a disease has been tracked for several years, we know its baseline rate. We do not expect a big change from year to year. If this happens, it triggers an investigation into the cause so we may intervene to prevent a worsening epidemic. In the mid 1980s, an alarming increase occurred in the incidence of tuberculosis (Figure 1-3) which alerted health care officials to an impending epidemic. Previously it seemed that tuberculosis was on its way to being suppressed in the United States because of the public health efforts that were in effect to control it. The increased incidence was partially attributed to the emergence of human immunodeficiency virus (HIV) infection, which increases one's susceptibility to tuberculosis. This observation led to increased efforts to identify the affected individuals and ensure that they were treated.

Prevalence, on the other hand, is the number of persons affected with a disease compared to the number of persons in the population who could have the disease, at any given time. It does not account for the duration of the disease. It is like looking

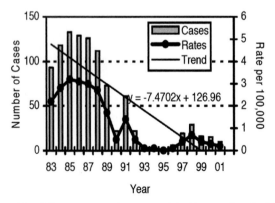

FIGURE 1-1 *Hemophilus influenzae*-caused cases and incidence rates, Louisiana, 1983–2001. *(From www.oph.dhh.louisiana.gov)*

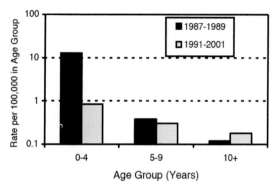

FIGURE 1-2 Diseases caused by *Hemophilus influenzae,* average annual incidence rates by age and time period, Louisiana, 1987–1989 and 1991–2000. *(From www.oph.dhh.louisiana.gov)*

at a slice of the population at a point in time to see who has the disease and who does not. Since it does not identify the new cases, it is not a measure of risk, but it does reflect the burden of disease on the community.

- *Prevalence is the number of affected persons divided by the total individuals at a point in time.*

The prevalence of diabetes shown in Figure 1-4 includes all adults who have been diagnosed with this disease compared to the number in the population, expressed as a percentage. As of 2000, the total number of diabetics in the United States was a staggering 17 million (6.2% of the population), which included an estimate of those who were undiagnosed. We could also look at the prevalence of diabetes in other groups, such as those who are on dialysis for renal failure. In this case the denominator would not be the entire population; it would be all those with end-stage renal disease (ESRD). Knowing the prevalence of a disease allows us to provide adequate health

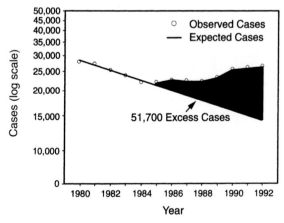

FIGURE 1-3 Expected and observed number of tuberculosis cases, United States, 1980–1992. *(From Centers for Disease Control and Prevention. 1993. MMWR, 42:696.)*

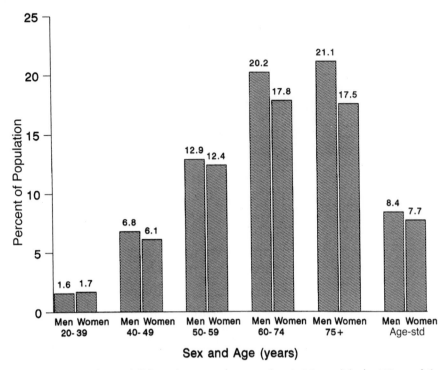

FIGURE 1-4 Prevalence of diabetes in men and women (age > 20 years) in the U.S. population. Diabetes includes previously diagnosed and undiagnosed disease, defined by fasting plasma glucose > 126 mg/dl; age is standardized. *(From Colwell, J. A. 2003. Diabetes hot topics. Philadelphia: Hanley & Belfus, p. 2.)*

care services such as dialysis centers. It is also useful when making decisions on the distribution of health care funds.

Incidence and prevalence are related. One way to increase the prevalence of a disease is to add new cases. This, of course, means that there has been an increase in the incidence of a disease, which happens when more people meet the criteria for diagnosis. On occasion, the criteria to diagnose a given condition may change or intensive screening programs may pick up more individuals who meet criteria. This could also account for a change in incidence rates, resulting in increased prevalence as well.

Attrition, or decrease in prevalence, occurs when people are either cured or die. A steady state occurs when the incidence is equal to the attrition. The prevalence pot shown in Figure 1-5 is a delightful diagram that illustrates the relationship between incidence, prevalence, cure, and mortality. A decrease in prevalence could result from a successful prevention program that would result in a decrease in the incidence of new cases. Keep in mind, however, that a decrease in prevalence could also be due to excessive mortality of the affected persons.

On the other hand, when prevalence goes up, it may be due to increased incidence but it may also be due to other factors. Many diseases that are highly prevalent are not curable but can be managed medically over many years, so the number of people

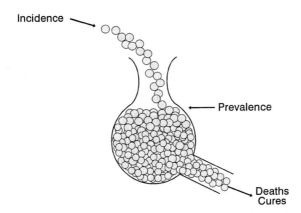

FIGURE 1-5 Relationship between incidence and prevalence: IV. *(From Gordis, L. 2004. Epidemiology, updated 3rd ed. Philadelphia: W.B. Saunders, p. 37.)*

with these diseases accumulates over time. Congestive heart failure, ESRD, vascular disease, and diabetes are a few examples. Even if preventive programs are successfully controlling the incidence of new cases, prevalence could increase because of better management and longer life spans of the affected persons. Whatever the cause, increased prevalence reflects a bigger societal burden, which translates into higher health care costs.

Types of Statistics

In general, there are two broad applications of statistics. A collection of data that describes the characteristics of the sample under study is called *descriptive statistics*. This type of database does not make conclusions using statistical tests. It is for informational purposes only.

- *Descriptive statistics is a set of observations that describe the characteristics of a sample.*

In the medical field, this may be used to outline an individual's (or institution's) experience with a certain type of pathology, such as the number or type of lung cancers diagnosed over a period of time. The data in Table 1-1 were compiled by the National Cancer Institute. They report the average annual incidence of lung cancers per 100,000 people diagnosed in men and women in different age groups. They reflect the risk that an average person will develop lung cancer in a given year.

We see that the incidence peaks in men at a later age (75–79) than in women (70–74), and the overall incidence of lung cancer is higher in men than women for the years that were studied. It is the nature of biologic data to spread over a range of values and peak at certain values, as we are seeing here. Note that this type of table does not tell us whether there is a *significant* gender difference in the incidence of lung cancer, or whether this experience is significantly different from the number of cancers in the general population during other years. These are descriptive data only. The numbers will ordinarily change from year to year, but to see whether an

TABLE 1-1 Annual Age-Specific Incidence Rates by Gender (per 100,000) for Cancers of the Lung and Bronchus

Age	Males	Females
0 to 4	0.00	0.00
5 to 9	0.00	0.00
10 to 14	0.00	0.80
15 to 19	0.15	0.12
20 to 24	0.16	0.23
25 to 29	0.46	0.56
30 to 34	1.76	1.26
35 to 39	5.40	4.15
40 to 44	21.59	14.46
45 to 49	51.31	31.84
50 to 54	104.60	56.94
55 to 59	198.15	89.97
60 to 64	283.17	123.10
65 to 69	380.18	142.84
70 to 74	459.64	153.08
75 to 79	469.67	135.20
80 to 84	441.69	108.03
85 and over	314.12	75.17

From Sondik, E. ed. (1988). *Annual Cancer Statistics Review*. Washington, D.C.: Division of Cancer Prevention and Control, National Cancer Institute. 1989.

intervention (such as an antismoking campaign) has a significant beneficial effect would require further collection of data over many years, given the long lag time between the exposure to cigarettes and the development of lung cancer. To make the comparison, you would need to perform a statistical test that compares the data.

Inferential statistics, on the other hand, does just that. It applies mathematical formulas to the data to make comparisons between two or more groups.

- *Inferential statistics uses data from a sample to make comparisons and draw conclusions about a larger group that the sample represents.*

One fundamental application of clinical research is to identify a particular pathway or intervention that will benefit a group of people. The initial assembly is divided into groups, as shown in Figure 1-6, and each group is exposed to a different pathway or treatment. At the end of the trial, the effect of each treatment is measured in the groups. For instance, to compare a new surgical intervention to the standard medical treatment for lung cancer, you could randomly assign lung cancer patients to receive either treatment, and compare mortality rates after a period of time.

By comparing the results, inferential statistics can tell us whether one pathway showed a significant advantage. Different formulas are used to answer different types of questions but the same reasoning is behind each statistical test. It is necessary to know when and how to use these formulas if you are going to be analyzing the data yourself.

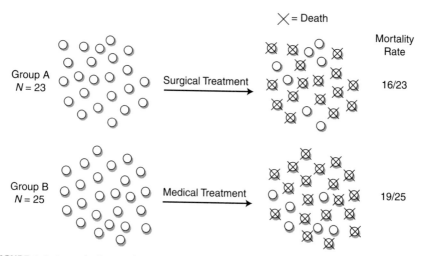

FIGURE 1-6 A standard type of research protocol where each group is exposed to a different treatment and the end result is compared after a period of time.

However, most researchers rely on statisticians to apply the appropriate formulas to their data. If you understand the common logic behind inferential statistics, you will be able to interpret any type of study.

KEY POINTS

- Diseases tend to cluster in groups of people.
- Epidemiology is the study of the spread of disease in a population.
- Measurements of disease in a population are necessary to follow trends, identify epidemics, and assess prevention and treatment programs.
- Incidence is the number of new cases of a disease divided by the number of people at risk for the disease, over a given period of time. Because it measures an event over time, it is expressed as a rate.
- Incidence is a measure of risk of getting the disease over a period of time for each member of the population.
- Incidence is used to track baseline rates of disease and to measure the effectiveness of prevention programs.
- Prevalence is the number of affected persons divided by the total population at a point in time.
- Prevalence reflects the burden of the disease on the community.
- Prevalence goes up with increased incidence or successful management programs which lengthen life spans.
- Prevalence decreases with excessive mortality, cures, or successful preventive programs.
- Descriptive statistics describes the characteristics of a data set taken from a sample.
- Inferential statistics makes comparisons and draws conclusions about a larger group based on the sample data.

REFERENCE

1. Gordis, L. 2004. *Epidemiology,* Philadelphia PA: WB Saunders.

REVIEW QUESTIONS

1. Rate and risk refer to the number of _____ that happen over time.

2. Incidence is the number of _____ cases of a disease that appear over time.

3. Incidence is a _____ and a measure of _____.

4. Prevalence is the number of cases of a disease at a _____ in time.

5. The graph in Figure 1-4 shows the prevalence of diabetes in different age groups. This is an example of _____ statistics.

6. To detect a significant difference in the prevalence of diabetes among different age groups would require _____ statistics.

7. If incidence increases and all other things are equal, prevalence _____.

8. If mortality increases and all other things are equal, prevalence _____.

9. As management improves life span in chronic disease, the prevalence _____.

ANSWERS TO REVIEW QUESTIONS

1. events

2. new

3. rate, risk

4. point

5. descriptive

6. inferential

7. increases

8. decreases

9. increases

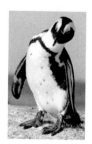

CHAPTER 2

Mathematical Principles

Our lives teem with numbers, but we sometimes forget that numbers are only tools.

—*Peter L. Bernstein*[1]

A common application of inferential biostatistics uses comparisons to see whether one pathway is better than another. A sample is selected and divided into groups. The groups are exposed to different interventions and the end results for each group are observed and compared. The result, such as mortality rate, is expressed as a numerical value. So, by definition, some math is involved. The math you need to know, however, is basic and involves comparisons in the form of ratios or simple algebraic formulas. A review of these concepts and a discussion of the various types of graphs you are likely to encounter are presented in this chapter.

RATIOS

When comparisons are made between the proportion of an attribute in two or more groups, the proportions are often expressed as ratios, such as the mortality ratio of persons treated with medical therapy versus those with surgical therapy. Ratios result from the comparison of fractions. Every fraction has a numerator, N, and a denominator, D.

$$\frac{N}{D}$$

D reflects the number of subjects in the group, such as the number of subjects getting standard medical treatment. N is the number of subjects with the characteristic being measured in the group, such as mortality. Figure 2-1 illustrates the results of a study where subjects with lung cancer received either medical or surgical treatment and mortality rates were compared.

It is easier to compare fractions when the denominator of each fraction is the same. This is done by converting the fractions so the denominators are expressed as equal values. Multiplying the numerator and the denominator by the same number does not change the value of the fraction (this is because you are essentially multiplying the fraction by 1). The ratios can be compared by the value of the numerators.

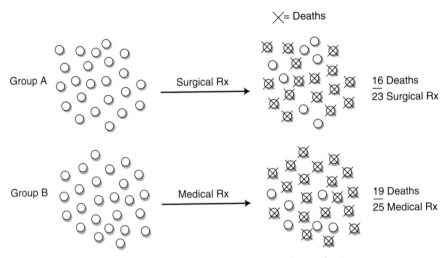

FIGURE 2-1 The mortality rates of each group can be compared using fractions.

For example, group A had 16 deaths out of 23 individuals in 5 years. Group B had 19 deaths out of 25 individuals in the same time period. Which group fared worse?

$$\frac{16}{23} \text{ compared to } \frac{19}{25}$$

This problem is easier to solve if there are equal denominators. We multiply the first fraction by 25/25 and the second fraction by 23/23 to convert to equal denominators, without changing the value of the individual fractions.

$$\text{Group A } \frac{16}{23} \times \frac{25}{25} = \frac{400}{575}$$

$$\text{Group B } \frac{19}{25} \times \frac{23}{23} = \frac{437}{575}$$

Group B did worse; they had a higher death rate.

Another way to compare ratios is to reduce each fraction so that the denominator is equal to 1. Any numerator over a denominator of 1 equals itself. (It follows that any number is actually itself divided by 1.) Do this by dividing the numerator by the denominator. When all fractions in a group are reduced so that their denominators are equal (such as 1 or 100), it is legitimate to compare numerators.

$$\text{Group A } \frac{16}{23} = 0.70$$

$$\text{Group B } \frac{19}{25} = 0.76$$

Again, we see that group B had a higher mortality rate.

Fractions can also be expressed as percentages. This implies that the denominators have all been converted to 100. It is easy to compare relative values using the percentage scale, since our currency is based on 100 and all of us know how to compare prices!

$$\text{Group A} \quad \frac{16}{23} = 0.70$$

$$\text{Group B} \quad \frac{19}{25} = 0.76$$

$$\text{Group A} \quad \frac{16}{23} \times 100 = 70\%$$

$$\text{Group B} \quad \frac{19}{25} \times 100 = 76\%$$

Group A had a 70% mortality rate, whereas Group B had a 76% mortality rate.

We can combine the mortality rates for two groups into one number known as a ratio. The mortality rate of one group becomes the numerator, N, and the mortality rate of the other group becomes the denominator, D. Both the numerator and denominator are fractions in themselves. For our purposes, when one fraction is divided by another, this will be designated by a double line. Dividing the two mortality rates results in a single number, the mortality ratio.

$$\frac{\dfrac{16}{23}}{\dfrac{19}{25}} = 0.92$$

It is not always apparent which group was designated to be in the numerator and which was designated as the denominator. If the result is less than 1, we know that the mortality rate of the group represented in the numerator was less than the other group, but we often need to rely on an explanation in the text to identify exactly which group fared better.

2 × 2 TABLES

One common method of displaying the data that measures the prevalence of a characteristic in each of two groups is a chart known as a 2 × 2 table. These tables can be confusing at first glance because it is intuitive to give the four boxes equal emphasis, but actually they should be interpreted in a sequence. For the above example, the cells hold the number of subjects who died versus those remaining alive after the study period.

	Dead	Alive
Group A	16	7
Group B	19	6

First, identify the groups being compared by imagining a double line. We need to add the rows the get the total number in each group. These will be the denominators.

	Dead	Alive	
Group A	16	7	**23**
Group B	19	6	**25**

Then identify the numerator, which is the characteristic being measured. This example is comparing mortality rates, so the number of deceased subjects for each group will be the numerators.

Group A	⑯	7	㉓	$\dfrac{16}{23}$	
Group B	⑲	6	㉕	$\dfrac{19}{25}$	= 0.92

The 2 × 2 table is extremely common. Like the basic black dress, it is ideal for many different situations. (It is very simple in construction, yet elegant in the way it shows off its figures!) There are several applications of this type of data display, and you will undoubtedly encounter this table many times. Remember to interpret these data by first identifying the groups or denominators.

LOGIC AND VENN DIAGRAMS

Certain groups of individuals tend to have associated characteristics. For instance, people with diabetes tend to have end-stage renal disease (ESRD) requiring dialysis. But not all people on dialysis have diabetes, and not all diabetics have renal failure. These relationships can be expressed graphically as Venn diagrams, where one circle represents condition 1 and another circle represents condition 2. An example of a Venn diagram is shown in Figure 2-2. These are rough diagrams that do not have numerical meaning, but the relative sizes of the circles are often a crude estimate of

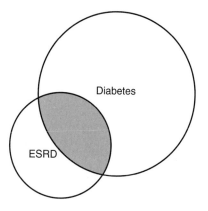

FIGURE 2-2 The crude relationship between diabetes and ESRD. We see that the prevalence of diabetes is higher than ESRD, and that roughly half of those with ESRD have diabetes. *(After Arkey, R. A., consulting ed. 2001. MKSAP 12: Nephrology and hypertension. Philadelphia: American College of Physicians-American Society of Internal Medicine).*

the relative prevalence of the conditions. The overlap represents those subjects with both conditions.

Venn diagrams do not need to be limited to two conditions. For example, Figure 2-3 illustrates the relationship between asthma, chronic bronchitis, and emphysema. Some people have just one of these conditions, others have two, and the ones represented in the middle of the diagram have been diagnosed with all three. This Venn diagram also illustrates that none of these conditions is exclusive. The presence of one condition does not exclude the possibility of having another.

Venn diagrams are used to illustrate an early awareness between connected conditions. As one circle encroaches upon another or the overlap increases, we may be prompted to perform further observational tests to try to quantify that relationship.

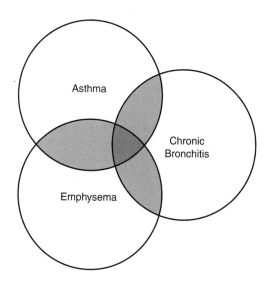

FIGURE 2-3 Asthma, chronic bronchitis, and emphysema can occur singly, as two conditions in one individual, or all three together.

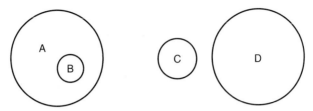

FIGURE 2-4 In the first diagram, the B circle is inside of A. Having the characteristic of A is a necessary requirement to also have B. The second diagram illustrates mutually exclusive conditions, where having one condition (represented by C) excludes you from having the other (represented by D).

In fact, as we continue to learn more about diseases and their epidemiology, such Venn diagrams are revised.

When one circle is completely within another bigger circle, as in Figure 2-4, everyone with the condition represented by the smaller circle will also have the other condition as well. This is an example of an inclusive condition where you must have condition A if you have condition B. These are more unusual, since most conditions have at least a few exceptions to the rule. On the other hand, mutually exclusive conditions have two separate circles that do not touch (circles C and D). Having one condition excludes you from having the other.

The Venn diagram in Figure 2-5 describes the relationship between atherosclerotic coronary artery disease (ACAD) and the presence of one or more risk factors of hypertension, diabetes, hyperlipidemia, or family history of ACAD.

Venn diagrams can be very telling when they are used to describe relationships which may be laced with bias. For instance, the early psychiatric research that was done on homosexuals assumed that they all had a mental disorder. In fact, up until 1973, the *Diagnostic and Statistical Manual of Mental Disorders* published by the American Psychiatric Association listed homosexuality as a disease, and treatment centered around "converting" these individuals to a heterosexual orientation.[2] The Venn diagram that represents this perception would look like Figure 2-6.

This diagram represents the belief that *all* homosexuals are mentally ill. However, we now know that many homosexuals are socially well-adjusted and comfortable

FIGURE 2-5 This Venn diagram shows that ACAD is overwhelmingly linked to risk factors because the ACAD circle is almost completely encompassed by the risk factor circle. Almost everyone with ACAD has at least one risk factor, although there are many people walking around with one or more risk factors who do not have ACAD. There are very few cases of people with ACAD who have none of these risk factors. It should be noted that this diagram does not indicate that risk factors *cause* ACAD, only that there is an observed association.

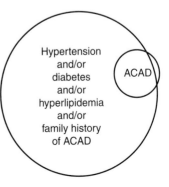

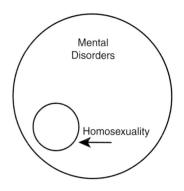

FIGURE 2-6 A Venn diagram describing a relationship laced with bias.

with their orientation. Psychiatrists failed to realize that they were not looking at the whole denominator of homosexuals when classifying this condition as a disease. The homosexuals they encountered were referred for a psychiatric illness, but that did not mean that *all* homosexuals had a psychiatric disorder. Many homosexuals had no mental impairment and therefore had no reason to seek psychiatric counseling. It took years of efforts on behalf of these individuals to change the classification (and, hence, the Venn diagram) into something like Figure 2-7.

This is a much different picture! The psychiatrists who originally classified homosexuality as a mental disorder were not accounting for all the facts, but they may have also been influenced by social and religious bias against homosexuals. Venn diagrams can be used to represent objective observations but could also reflect associations that are subject to bias. It is an easy jump to form a generalization about a profession, religion, or race based on a few observations. Always keep in mind the possibility of a bigger circle when making judgments and forming opinions. There may be a so-called silent majority that has not been accounted for. Never underestimate the true denominator. This is a good practice to apply in both our professional lives and our social interactions. Consider the situation described in Box 2-1.

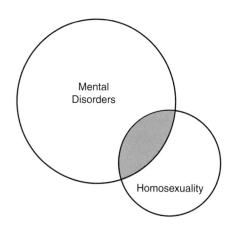

FIGURE 2-7 A Venn diagram with changed classifications to reverse an old belief that all homosexuals are mentally ill.

BOX 2-1

I recently had a discussion with a house officer who had spent the morning evaluating patients admitted to the Emergency Department (ED) the night before with chest pain. He was frustrated at the number of patients admitted with apparently noncardiac causes of their pain. He commented that the ED physicians admit everyone who presents with chest pain. Draw the Venn diagram of his perception of group P (those who present to the ED with chest pain) and group A (those who get admitted with chest pain). Assume all admissions for chest pain come through the ED.

All those who present (group P) get admitted (group A). Therefore, group P is contained entirely within group A. On the other hand, do all who get admitted with chest pain (group A) present to ER with chest pain (group P)? If we assume that all the admissions come through the ED, then group A will be contained within group P. The two circles will be superimposed.

Now draw the Venn diagram for the perception of the physician who was actually working the night shift in the ED for presenters (P) and admits (A). I suspect that group P will be larger than group A. There may have been several patients who were evaluated for chest pain and released, unbeknownst to the house officer.

RELATIONSHIPS AMONG CHARACTERISTICS

The value of one characteristic will frequently be linked to another in a constant way that can be expressed numerically. For instance, level of education is linked to yearly income: people with more schooling generally make more money.

This numerical relationship can be expressed in three ways:

1. *Words.* We can make a statement about the strength of the relationship. For instance, we might say that every additional year of post-high school training increases income by a certain average amount, such as $10,000, in addition to a base income which might be $30,000 (these are fictitious data).

2. *Formulas.* These are more intellectually satisfying but require the reader to understand the symbols that are used. For instance, the familiar formula $y = bx + a$ represents a linear association between y (the *dependent* variable) and x (the *independent* variable). y depends on the value of x. The strength of the effect that x has on y is reflected in the value of b. a is known as the y-intercept, or the baseline value of y when $x = 0$. Using the income example, the independent variable x is the number of post-high school years of training, and b is the effect on income of each year of additional training. The baseline income of $30,000 for those with no training beyond high school is represented by a. The average yearly income is represented by y, which depends on the value of x, added to the baseline income.

When we need to know multiple values of y, it may be easier to consult a table that has already solved the equation for different values of x. One common example of this is a table that converts temperature from Fahrenheit into Celsius. We will also see several examples of statistical tables that take a variety of values and convert them into probabilities.

3. *Graphs.* This is the most informative way to display a relationship between variables. These easily convey the type and strength of relationship that exists between values. It is more enlightening to see an illustration rather than trying to interpret verbal or numerical descriptors.

- *The x-axis is the abscissa.*
- *The y-axis is the ordinate.*

The graph in Figure 2-8 shows that the amount that *y* increases depends on the value of *b*, which is the *slope* of the line.

How to Read a Graph: A Stepwise Approach

Even though this seems rudimentary, it is a good habit to go through these simple steps in sequence whenever you come across a graph. Learn to do this every time.

1. *Look at the title.* Surprisingly, many of us do this last because we are drawn to the pictorial display of the data. It is much more efficient to focus first on the content of the graph before looking at the plot. Sometimes you need to search for the title. It may be in the caption, as in Figure 2-9. On occasion, you may find it only in the text.
2. *Look at the label on the abscissa (x-axis).* This represents the independent variable. This variable may be plotted in a continuous fashion. Alternatively, the abscissa may represent different groups, as in a bar graph.
3. *Look at the label on the ordinate (y-axis).* This is called the dependent variable. Pay attention to the range of values, since they may not represent what you would intuitively think. Some values may have been excluded from the range, especially if only a few data points live there. The graph of average yearly income (Figure 2-8) could be displayed without the lower levels of income since they were redundant in our example.

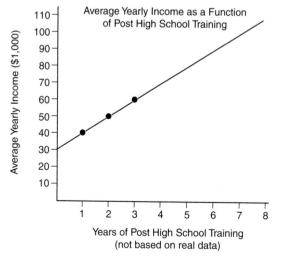

FIGURE 2-8 The graph for the equation $y = 10,000\,x + 30,000$. For every unit increase in x, y increases by 10,000. The y-intercept is 30,000.

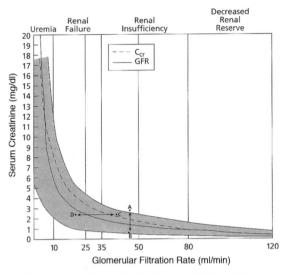

FIGURE 2-9 Relationships between glomerular filtration rate (GFR) by ^{125}I-iothalamate clearance and serum creatinine concentration and stage of chronic kidney disease.

4. *Look at the line or bar that defines the relationship.* This is the meat of the graph. It is easier to interpret it after going through the prior steps. Some graphs contain a lot of information and may show several relationships in one picture, using different lines or multiple colored bars to represent different groups. Note that when *x* is plotted in a continuous fashion, the slope of the line represents the effect that *x* has on *y*. If it is a straight line, *x* has a constant effect on *y*. If the line is curved, the magnitude of the effect on *y* changes with the value of *x*, as in the equation: $y = x^2$.
5. Draw your own conclusions. This is like the dessert! It is the summation of the prior steps. Compare your conclusions with that of the author(s). Figure 2-9 may seem a little confusing at first glance. Let us look at it using this stepwise approach.

First find the title (in this case, it is in the caption). It helps to know that the glomerular filtration rate (GFR) is a direct reflection of kidney function, and that the most accurate way to measure GFR is by injecting a substance known as ^{125}I-iothalamate and then measuring the volume of blood that the kidneys are able to clear of this substance in 1 minute. Since this is a very cumbersome method, it is not used in medical practice. A much simpler method is to do a blood test measuring serum creatinine. This graph represents a relationship between the GFR measured by the highly accurate ^{125}I-iothalamate and the serum creatinine. It is essentially a comment on the reliability of creatinine for estimating kidney function.

Next, note that the abscissa is plotted in continuous values, from 0 ml/min (no kidney function) to 120 ml/min. Is this the absolute best kidney function? Probably not, but values higher than this would not give any further information. The GFR has been subdivided into levels of renal function, but the groups are not equal. "Uremia" and "Failure" have a smaller range of values. The divisions get smaller at lower levels of GFR as the creatinine starts to rise rapidly. This may help to identify people who have severe disease before they actually have kidney failure.

The ordinate contains values for serum creatinine. The values cut off at 20 mg/dl, but anything above this value would not enhance the message.

What is the relationship? Notice that there are two lines encompassing a gray area, implying that there are data points between these lines. This means there is a range of creatinine values for a given GFR in different people, and that the range gets really wide as the GFR declines. Also note that the lines are curved. The effect of kidney function on the serum creatinine level is not linear. As GFR falls, the creatinine initially manifests very little change. At the lower levels of kidney function, it can go up dramatically.

So what is the conclusion? Points A and B in Figure 2-9 represent the range of creatinine that could be seen in a group of individuals with the same kidney function. At a normal GFR the range is very tight. At lower levels of kidney function, however, there is an extremely wide range of observed creatinine values. Other factors that affect serum creatinine have a much bigger influence as kidney function falls.

Points C and D in Figure 2-9 show how individuals with different levels of kidney filtering ability can still have the same creatinine levels. The authors explain this by differences in muscle mass, which accounts for most of the creatinine in the blood. As kidney function fails, creatinine builds up. In fact, when estimating GFR, formulas are used that include not only serum creatinine but also other factors that account for muscle mass such as height, weight, gender, and sometimes race. This point might be better emphasized by lowering point D to 1.5 mg/dl and placing point C in a parallel position in Renal Insufficiency category.

Overall, the use of serum creatinine to estimate kidney function is very helpful. A creatinine value greater than 2 mg/dl should raise suspicion of at least moderate kidney disease. These data points represent a large number of individuals at a given point in time, but do not tell what happens to an individual's creatinine values as renal failure progresses. Could one track the serum creatinine over time in a given individual to monitor renal function, or would the range of values vary too much to be useful? (In fact, it *is* very useful to monitor serum creatinine over time for an individual, although this graph does not give that information.)

Do you agree with the above conclusions?

MATHEMATICAL EQUATIONS AND DATA

One of the applications of mathematics is to solve equations. When we are given the values of one variable, we can solve for the value of another, as in $y = bx + a$. When we deal with data, however, we start with the values of x and y for each subject and we try to find the equation that best describes the relationship. This is particularly challenging because the values we see in nature do not adhere to a strict mathematical relationship. For any value of x, there will be more than one value of y because of the natural variability of biologic data. For instance, is there an association between height and weight? If each subject is measured for height and weight, we see that not all subjects with the same height will weigh the same. If a relationship does exist, however, we try to define the model that has the best fit for the observations we have.

- *Statistics uses observations to define mathematical relationships.*

KEY POINTS

- Fractions can be compared when their denominators are expressed as equal values. If a fraction represents the end result of an intervention in each group, the fractions can be compared and reported as a single value or ratio.
- 2×2 tables organize data into groups, and display the frequency of a characteristic within each group.
- Venn diagrams are used to show crude associations between characteristics.
- Always consider the entire denominator when looking at data or making judgments.
- When characteristics are related numerically, the best way to describe this is with a graph.
- The x-axis is the abscissa.
- The y-axis is the ordinate.
- Learn how to read a graph in a stepwise fashion:
  1. Read the title to orient yourself.
  2. Identify the units on the abscissa.
  3. Identify the units on the ordinate.
  4. Note the relationship between the plotted points.
  5. Draw your own conclusions.
- Statistics uses observations to try to find the best mathematical model to describe a relationship.

REFERENCES

1. Bernstein, P. L. 1998. *Against the gods.* New York: John Wiley & Sons, Inc., p. 7.
2. Kaplan, B. J. and V. A. Sadock. 2000. *Comprehensive textbook of psychiatry.* Philadelphia: Lippincott, Williams & Wilkins.

REVIEW QUESTIONS

1. A _____ is one way to report a comparison in mortality rates as a single number.

2. Two different medical regimens were compared for breast cancer. The mortality ratio was 1.23. The group that fared better was in the _____ of the ratio calculation.

3. A study that reports a mortality ratio of 1 shows that the groups had _____ mortality rates.

4. Venn diagrams are a way of illustrating _____ relationships among characteristics.

5. The solutions to an equation for multiple values of an independent variable can sometimes be found in a _____.

6. When you read a graph, look at the _____ and _____ of the abscissa and ordinate before you interpret the relationship between the variables so you can put the data into proper context.

7. Observations in nature do not adhere to a strict _____ equation, but we try to find the best model that describes the relationship.

ANSWERS TO REVIEW QUESTIONS

1. ratio

2. denominator

3. equal

4. crude

5. table

6. units, scale

7. mathematical

CHAPTER **3**

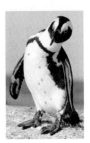

Populations

Population: 1. The total number of persons inhabiting a country, city or any district. 2. The body of inhabitants of a place. 3. The assemblage of organisms under consideration. 4. An aggregate of statistical items.

—*The American College Dictionary*[1]

Statisticians think in terms of large numbers. They focus on the multitude rather than the individual. Once you make this transition, you will be on your way to understanding the theory behind biostatistics and the process of inference.

THEORETICAL CONCEPTS OF POPULATIONS

Most of us deal almost exclusively with individual situations throughout the day. The recommendations we make to patients depend upon the particulars of their condition. Through the formal education process, we have been trained to respond in a certain way in a given situation. Our actions are further influenced by our personal experience and some of us have accumulated quite an extensive and valuable collection.

The theory behind biostatistics expands on this principle. Imagine being able to observe the response to a given treatment (through a totally unbiased approach) of *not just one* patient, but of an *infinite* number of patients. Not all patients would have the same outcome. However, the results would tend to cluster and, if the treatment helped, the outcome would be better overall than with a different pathway that did not work as well. Armed with this extensive knowledge, you could make a prediction for an individual result based on the responses observed in the larger group.

We usually think of populations in terms of people who occupy a certain piece of land but, in statistical language, the definition is actually much broader. When we encounter the medical literature, the populations studied are usually groups of people with common, quantifiable characteristics. (Some statistics textbooks define populations as collections of data or observations. This refers to the actual data set taken from the collection of units or things being studied. For our purposes, we will use the more universal definition of populations as collections of the units themselves.)

- *A population is a collection of things having some quantifiable characteristic in common.*

We identify populations based on what we would like to study. A population could be composed of just about anything. It could be wine grapes harvested from a certain county which we would like to taste-test. It could be springs produced in a factory, of which we would like to test the tensile strength. It could be insect eggs or raindrops. It could be children with asthma or women with osteoporosis.

A true population is a theoretical concept. In theory, many populations cannot be counted completely since the number in the collection is extremely large. Take the example of raindrops. If we consider not only all raindrops that are falling at the current time but also those that have fallen in the past, and those yet to come, the true number approaches infinity. Many populations are so huge that it is impossible to account for each member, such as patients with congestive heart failure. A Venn diagram of a large population might have indistinct, muted edges or arrows pointing concentrically away from the center, as in Figure 3-1.

It is widely accepted to use a distinct circle to represent a population. When you see a traditional circle that represents a large population, try to think in terms of these concepts.

Another reason why populations do not have crisp edges is that, in many cases, they are constantly changing. Think of the population of kids with asthma. The definition of asthma is firm. In other words, the members of the population share a measurable characteristic, such as a collection of recurrent symptoms or the results of a breathing test. This is how we define the population. However, the members of the population are difficult to count at any given time. We set up criteria to distinguish members of the population, but new members are meeting these criteria every day while others are being disqualified. For example, new diagnoses of asthma are continually being made, which adds to the population. On the other hand, because children grow, there will be a continuous flux out of the population at whatever age (in minutes, perhaps seconds?) a "child" becomes "not a child."

POPULATION PARAMETERS

Every population has attributes we attempt to measure. These are not the same as the characteristics that define the population, although the characteristics and attributes may overlap. The attributes are referred to as *parameters*. Even though populations are fluid, their attributes are quite stable. For instance, consider the parameter of "average age" in the population of U.S. citizens. If you were able to measure the average age of the population of the United States, it would not vary from day to day, even though many people enter this population through birth and immigration, and many exit through death and change of citizenship. The flux of people entering and exiting the population has a negligible effect on average age. Although populations

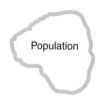 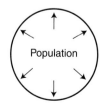

FIGURE 3-1. Venn diagrams of large populations with indistinct, muted edges and arrows pointing concentrically away from the center.

in themselves can be immeasurable entities, they are very real and their parameters are unyielding. There *is* an average age of the U.S. population and it does not vary over days or even several weeks, although it may shift gradually over years.

A parameter may be something simple to grasp, like average age. It could also be something more abstract, like the risk of an accident in a population of drunken drivers or the survival rate in a population of people with a certain type of cancer. A population parameter is numerically very solid. We may not be able to know it exactly but we can estimate it with a degree of certainty, using statistical techniques.

The fact that the population attributes or parameters are firm is a very important concept in biostatistics. Consider the parameter of risk of an accident in a population of drunken drivers. We could define the population by the common characteristic of a blood alcohol level greater than a certain cutoff point. The population is further defined by those meeting the above blood alcohol criterion who are behind the wheel of a moving vehicle. You may recognize this as a population that is constantly changing. Individuals enter and exit this population all the time. There is no way to account for all of them at any one point.

The parameter of *risk* is a number that has a concrete value. It is the chance of an impaired driver having an accident within a unit of time when he or she is on the road. The risk exists and it is a fixed value, even though the population is fluid (in more ways than one!). We cannot exactly measure this risk but we can estimate it using observations. The point being made here is that any parameter of a population is *stable* and, although we may not have access to the exact number, we have the methods to estimate it using observations.

- *A population parameter is a numerical value that summarizes the population data.*

This is not to say that we cannot change that risk. In fact, that is one of the quintessential applications of biostatistics: to decrease the risk of a bad outcome in a given situation. Drunk drivers have a higher risk of accidents than do sober ones, so we have increased public awareness of this problem and have enacted laws to discourage people from driving in this condition. Safer cars have been designed to reduce the risk of morbidity and mortality when an accident does occur.

PRACTICAL CONCEPTS OF POPULATIONS

A population is defined as a collection of things having some quantifiable characteristic in common. Actually, the members of a population may (and often do) share more than one common characteristic. These should be quantifiable (i.e., there should be a reasonable way of distinguishing whether or not an individual possesses this characteristic).

For example, we may want to study the effect of a new anticancer agent on a group of people with a certain type of cancer. We would define our population as people with this type of cancer. The members of the population should be shown to have this quantifiable characteristic (they have this type of cancer) by a diagnosis made from a biopsy taken by a pathologist. We may want to exclude those with widespread disease if we think they might not respond as well to the treatment. If a favorable response is observed in our experiment, we may study those with metastatic disease at a later time. For now, we could exclude them from the population.

In clinical trials, populations are defined by *inclusion* and *exclusion* criteria. These criteria can be very stringent since the results may be muddied if there is too much variation in the characteristics of the members of the population. For instance, if subjects with different types of leukemia were included in our population, we may miss the fact that the new agent may be effective against a certain type of leukemia, since the overall effect would be diluted among the other subjects. Financial and other resources need to be considered as well. If the proposed trial is too inclusive, the cost of running the trial may be prohibitive.

On the other hand, if the exclusion criteria are too stringent we may not be able to enroll enough subjects who meet all the established criteria, or it may take too long to find the subjects needed. There is also the possibility of missing a potential effect on a subset of patients who might have responded if they had not originally been excluded.

As you can see, it can be quite challenging to even identify the population that is to be studied. In practice, populations are often described based on who is likely to respond to treatment. This information is taken from prior observations or pilot studies. If the condition being studied is prevalent, then subject enrollment is facilitated. As long as adequate funding is available, the population may be expanded by relaxing the exclusion criteria. A larger number of subjects allows us to study the effect of the treatment on subsets of patients after the results are in. Refer to the case study in Box 3-1.

BOX 3-1

The Heart Outcomes Prevention Evaluation (HOPE) Study investigators studied the effect of the antihypertensive agent ramipril on a population of people with cardiovascular disease or diabetes.[2] This drug works through a hormonal pathway. It was shown in prior studies to have beneficial effects in people with poor pumping function (known as heart failure) by preventing heart attacks. The investigators altered this population to study those with normal pump function.

Inclusion and Exclusion Criteria

- *Men and women at least 55 years old.*
- *History of coronary artery disease, stroke, peripheral vascular disease, or diabetes plus at least one of these: hypertension, elevated total cholesterol, low high-density lipoprotein (HDL) cholesterol, cigarette smoking, or microalbuminuria.*
- *No heart failure.*
- *Not taking angiotensin-converting enzyme inhibitor.*
- *Not taking vitamin E.*
- *No uncontrolled hypertension.*
- *No overt nephropathy.*
- *No prior myocardial infarction or stroke within 4 weeks.*

Cardiovascular disease and diabetes are prevalent, so the enrollment of 9297 patients who also met the other criteria was not surprising. Because of the large number of enrollees, the effect of the drug could be studied on subsets of patients as well. This included 10 subgroups altogether, such as those with and without hypertension, diabetes, and prior heart attack. The results showed an overall beneficial effect on the subjects and on 9 out of 10 subgroups. This information is now being used to treat those patients who meet the criteria for the population that was studied.

UNIDENTIFIED CHARACTERISTICS

There will undoubtedly be characteristics in members of the population that are not identified. The inclusion and exclusion criteria do not account for *all* the possible characteristics. For instance, subjects who enroll in a cancer treatment trial may not be asked about their daily intake of vitamins, and this could vary substantially among the individuals. Could this influence the observed result? Theoretically, vitamins *could* make a difference in one's response to treatment.

If the two pathways in the trial were a pharmaceutical treatment versus a "naturally occurring" remedy, and if subjects were free to choose the pathway they preferred, those who take vitamins may prefer to take the natural substance. If this pathway proved superior to the pharmaceutical treatment, it could be the result of a vitamin instead of the substance being tested. In this case, the treatment would get credit for making the difference even though the result may have been partially due to a factor that was not considered.

The results could have gone the other way—the effect of a vitamin may have diminished the effect of the natural substance or additively caused a harmful toxicity. In this case, the pharmaceutical substance would have been erroneously declared to have treatment benefit over the natural substance, when in fact it was the vitamin (which was not accounted for) that affected the results.

The unidentified characteristics that could potentially affect the result are referred to as *confounders*. If the unaccounted factors are equally distributed in the groups, however, their effect is negated. When subjects are randomized into groups and do not get to decide which pathway to take, the unaccounted factors should be evenly distributed and their effect on the results should cancel out.

THE ART OF MEDICINE

It is very convenient when individual patients meet the population criteria for a landmark study. It is a no-brainer to apply the results of a well-designed study to the appropriate patients. There will be many occasions, however, when a treatment decision will need to be made for an individual who meets some, but not all, of the criteria which defined the population of a particular study. Another common occurrence is that the insurance company will not pay the cost of the drug that is studied, but will cover the cost of a cheaper substitute.

In general, it is not good science to extrapolate the results of a study to a patient who is not a member of the population that was defined. There is also a valid argument against prescribing a substitute drug and expecting the same results. This is where the *art* of practicing medicine comes into play. In these situations, good judgment and rational thinking are needed to advise patients. It helps to stay informed of the literature in your field of practice. It is also beneficial to include patients in a discussion of options. They should be encouraged to participate in their own treatment decisions and voice an opinion after you provide them with the available data. Let them know, however, that the results may not be completely transferable to their particular scenario.

In summary, biostatistics deals not with the individual, but with the masses. Distance yourself from the singular; learn to think *big*. Instead of an individual patient, think of hundreds of patients just like that one. You can then tap into this

BOX 3-2

An example that illustrates the forward revisions in medical thinking is taken from a recently published article on acute aortic dissection, a potentially life-threatening condition.[3] *A delay in diagnosis can have a deleterious effect on the individual's chance of survival. This entity has been recognized for centuries but the diagnosis can be elusive. The investigators studied the presenting symptoms in 464 patients with acute aortic dissection who were enrolled in a registry from 12 large referral centers in 6 countries.*

They discovered that many of the classic symptoms described in textbooks were not as prevalent as previously thought. The character of pain has classically been taught to be tearing or ripping, and migratory throughout the chest cavity. However, most subjects defined their pain as sharp and nonmigratory. In addition, other typical signs—decreased pulse, heart murmur, and abnormal chest radiograph—were often absent. Interestingly, many patients presented with loss of consciousness, a symptom that was previously underrated.

This information will undoubtedly be useful to clinicians in the future when evaluating a patient with acute chest pain or syncope. Textbooks will be rewritten as more reliable information is accrued. The symptoms previously considered classic will be replaced with a different profile based on recent evidence.

exploded experience and use it to your patient's advantage. Learn to rely on the literature to guide your decisions. This is not meant to diminish the human quality of practicing medicine but rather to distance you emotionally from the recommendations you give.

Above all, biostatistics implores us to *keep an open mind*. There is nothing wrong with changing recommendations as long as it is done in the patient's best interest. As new evidence is revealed, it should be incorporated into practice patterns. The best health care providers work in a very fluid environment and continually update their knowledge base. They keep in mind that the most reliable evidence usually comes from large populations of patients with the same characteristics as the individual they are treating. Consider the example in Box 3-2.

KEY POINTS

- A population is a collection of things having some quantifiable characteristic in common. There may be multiple characteristics.
- Populations are defined by their common characteristics, called inclusion criteria.
- Populations are also defined by the common characteristics they lack; these are known as exclusion criteria.
- Unmeasured characteristics in a population are important considerations in experimental design.
- The science of inferential statistics is based on studies of populations; the results can be applied to all individuals who belong to the population.
- Many populations are so large that we cannot account for all the members.
- Populations have attributes called parameters, which are numerical values that summarize the data. These are distinctly different from their quantifiable characteristics.

- Even though populations are fluid, their parameters are stable.
- Use caution when extrapolating the results of studies on a specific population to patients who do not meet all the inclusion and exclusion criteria.
- New evidence is continually used to update sources of medical information.

REFERENCES

1. *The American College Dictionary.* 1969. New York: Random House, Inc., p. 943.
2. The HOPE Study Investigators. 2000. Effect of an angiotensin-converting enzyme inhibitor, ramipril, on cardiovascular events in high-risk patients. *New Engl J Med*, 342:3, 145.
3. Hagan, P. G. et al. 2000. The International Registry of Acute Aortic Dissection. *JAMA*, 283:7, 897.

R E V I E W   Q U E S T I O N S

1. _____ are collections of people or things with common quantifiable characteristics.

2. _____ and _____ criteria define a population.

3. _____ characteristics could potentially influence the result of a study if not equally distributed among the groups.

4. Populations are a theoretical concept, but their _____ are very real and measurable.

5. If a patient who is a member of a population that was studied wants to substitute a cheaper drug for the one that was shown to have benefit, s/he should be told _____.

A N S W E R S   T O   R E V I E W   Q U E S T I O N S

1. Populations

2. Inclusion, exclusion

3. Unaccounted

4. parameters

5. not to expect the same results as the study. However, in many cases this can be done, depending on other available information.

CHAPTER **4**

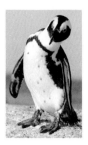

Samples

A basic characteristic of experimental science is the necessity for reaching conclusions on the basis of incomplete information.

—*M. Anthony Schork and Richard D. Remington*[1]

Populations may be based on theoretical concepts but the individual members that make up a population are very real. We need a way to concretely study a population that has been identified. As we have learned, populations can be very large; some have so many members that we cannot count them all. They are also very fluid, with a continuous flux of members that enter and exit. It is often impossible to study each individual member but this does not mean the endeavor of studying populations is futile. We use a method that relies on *sampling*.

A sample is a group of individuals that represents the population. If we choose the sample correctly, the results we get in the sample members will be very close to the results we would have gotten had we studied the whole population. The attribute being measured in the sample will approximate the value of that attribute in the entire population.

For instance, if we wanted to know the distribution of different religions in the United States, we could poll every person to find out their religious affiliation. This is, of course, an impossible task. If we choose a sample of people correctly, however, the proportions of different religions that we see in the sample would accurately reflect the proportions of different religions in the population.

SAMPLE SELECTION

Ideally, we choose a sample so there is equal representation of the individuals that comprise the population. That is to say, every member of the population has an equal chance of being chosen. This is called *random sampling*. The *law of independence* states that the choice of one member does not influence the chance of choosing any other. When sampling is done following the above rules, the laws of chance apply so that when we study the sample we know how close our observation will be to the real result we would observe had we studied the entire population. The numbers would not be exactly the same, however. For instance, the proportion of Baptists may be

10% in our sample whereas the real value in the population may be 12%. (These data are used as an example and are not based on actual studies.)

- *An independent, random sample is chosen in such a way that every possible combination of size N has an equal chance of being selected.*

If each individual in a population theoretically has an equal chance of being chosen for the sample, how many possible sample combinations of a given size *N* are there? If the population is large (as most are), then there is also an incredibly large number of possible combinations that could comprise the sample. For instance, in a smaller population of size 20, if we wanted to study a sample of size 5, there are 15,504 possible combinations! There is a formula to calculate this,* but the lesson to appreciate here is not how many possible different combinations of individuals could be chosen as the sample, but the fact that in a random, independent process each combination has an equally likely chance of being the sample.

It may seem that we are compromising our scientific methods by employing these sampling shortcuts to make life easy. When we use samples, we do not have access to the complete collection of information that we would ideally use if we studied the entire population, and we will not get an exact answer. We understand, however, the need to reach conclusions based on incomplete information. It is thus quite acceptable to study a population by using a sample as long as we accept a modicum of uncertainty in interpreting the results. We realize that by using samples we are actually estimating the result we would have gotten had we studied the entire population.

This is a vital point in biostatistics. It is important to consciously distinguish between populations and the samples that represent them. We refer to the attributes that characterize a population as *parameters*, in comparison to those observed in the sample, which are called *statistics*. In practice, we use sample statistics to estimate population parameters. In the above example regarding religion, the sample statistic of 10% Baptist is an estimate of the true population parameter of 12% Baptist (again, these are fictitious data).

- *The value of an attribute in a sample is called a statistic. A sample statistic is an estimate of the parameter, or true value, of that attribute in the population.*

ESTIMATES AND UNCERTAINTY

Since the sample statistic provides us with an estimate of the population parameter, it could be off in either direction. That is to say, the statistic could be an overestimation, an underestimation, or right on target. We don't know with certainty which of the above scenarios is right, but we are willing to accept a margin of error. When sample statistics are reported, they are often reported with their value plus or minus a certain amount. This range of values is called the *confidence interval*. These are like comfort zones that attempt to encompass the true population parameter. A narrow confidence interval means that our sample statistic is very likely to be a pretty close estimation of the population parameter.

---

*The formula is: $P!/N!\ (P-N)!$ where P = number in the population, N = number in the sample, and ! represents the act of multiplying the number consecutively by another number of descending value until 1 is reached.

- *The confidence interval is the sample statistic plus or minus the margin of error.*

The confidence interval is a range of values derived from the sample that has a given probability of encompassing the true value we seek. It reflects the margin of error that inherently goes along when we use sample statistics to estimate the true value of the population parameter. We will see how it is calculated but, for now, the important thing to know is that there is a given probability that the boundaries of the confidence interval contain the true population parameter.

It is customary to use a 5% degree of uncertainty in statistics. If the experiment were repeated over and over using different random samples of the same size, we would get a variety of results. There would be different estimates of the true parameter and each would have its own confidence interval.

Figure 4-1 represents the possible results that could occur if an experiment were repeated multiple times. The solid black line represents the true parameter, which is really unknown to us. Each confidence interval is encompassed by the brackets, with the sample statistic in the middle, designated by **X**. Overall, 95% (or 19 out of 20) of

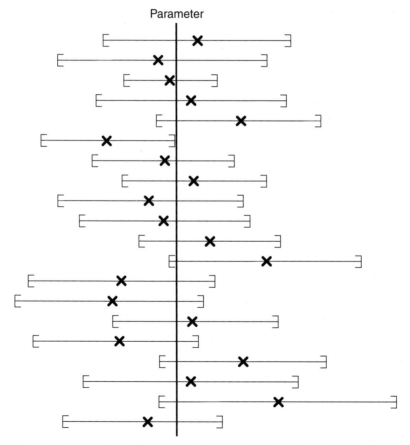

FIGURE 4-1 Twenty samples of the same size from a population. Each sample gives us a sample statistic represented by **X**. The boundaries of the confidence intervals are marked by brackets, [ ].

the confidence intervals will (in the long run) contain the true parameter. Since we only do the experiment once, any of these results could occur.

In the example using religious preference, we are not able to know the true percentage of 12% Baptist, but let us say that our sample statistic was 10% ± 3%. The confidence interval is thus 7% to 13%. We are not 100% sure that the confidence interval includes the actual parameter, but we are 95% sure if we followed the rules of random sampling and applied the correct statistical test. In this case, the confidence interval *does* include the true parameter (12% Baptist). Keep in mind, though, that we cannot know where the parameter actually lies in this interval. We can say with 95% certainty, however, that the interval ranging from 7% to 13% contains the true value.

It is intuitive to assume that a larger sample that has been randomly chosen from a population is more likely to give a more accurate result than a smaller one. In fact, this point is absolutely true. A larger sample will, on average, more accurately estimate the parameter and will have a narrower confidence interval because larger samples tend to have less overall variability of the characteristic being studied. There comes a point, however, where increasing a sample size will have diminishing returns. The investment of time, money, and inconvenience to the subjects will not offset the incremental degree of certainty that can be obtained from expanding the sample size. Ethical issues are brought up as well, since subjects participating in the experiments are accepting potential risk of being exposed to an unproven intervention. If the sample is larger than needed to obtain the answer we seek, why expose extra subjects to this unknown risk?

On the other hand, if a study has too few subjects it may not be able to detect a treatment difference if one does indeed exist. Statisticians can estimate the number of subjects needed to participate in an experiment once it has been designed. There is a formula (see Chapter 14) to calculate the minimum number of participants to obtain a *reasonably* reliable answer as to whether or not a particular pathway is better than another. Notice the word *reasonably* in the preceding sentence. We have said that investigators are comfortable with a small degree of uncertainty in estimating how a population would behave if all of its members could be observed. One of the elements that goes into the calculation for the sample size is the acceptable degree of uncertainty, usually 5%.

RANDOM SAMPLING AND ACCURACY

Consider the example in Box 4-1 regarding a quality issue on a production line. In order to test the tensile strength of a population of springs being produced in a factory, we use a random sample to see how many meet specifications. If each spring being produced has an equal chance of being a true representative of the variation in tensile strength, then taking a group of consecutively produced springs would be a fair representation of the population. However, there are many reasons why the value of the tensile strength could cluster during production. There may be a technician who is acutely attentive to production specs and the springs may be superior when that person is on the job, or there could be a variation in the machinery as the day progresses due to changing temperature of the equipment or the amount of lubricant in the moving parts. There may even be a difference in shifts, since midnight workers might get less sleep and thus be less observant.

BOX 4-1

Each of these circles represents the same population. The smaller circles represent individuals and the solid ones are individuals being asked to participate in a study. Which of these most appropriately represents random sampling?

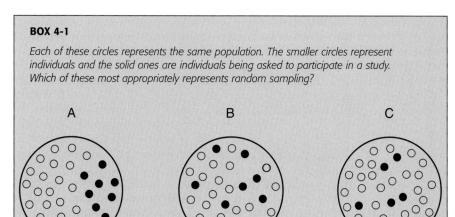

A   B   C

This is actually quite a tricky question. Let us think about this. The safest answer is B, which visually guarantees that the sample will represent diversity of the population. However, there is another thing to consider. If the members of the population are randomly distributed among themselves with respect to the characteristics being studied, then taking a chunk out of the population (as in A) will also represent a random sample. The problem is that in biostatistics the characteristics tend to cluster with regard to their value. The values are usually not randomly distributed. Baptists, like members of other religions, tend to cluster in certain regions. The pairs shown in diagram C would be subject to linkage, as well, which would violate the law of independence and would introduce bias into the results.

In this case, a sample of springs composed of those produced on all shifts and all days of the week would be more representative of the entire population. This example illustrates how an otherwise carefully designed study could result in an erroneous estimate of the population parameter due to an error in sampling. Published clinical studies should describe the method of sampling used. When reading this section of a study report, be aware that the sample might not truly represent the population.

EXTERNAL AND INTERNAL VALIDATION

It is customary to enroll subjects in studies as they present to larger referral centers where these studies are likely to be done. This is often done on a consecutive basis. If the subjects meet the study criteria, they are asked to participate, one after the other. If the patients are not connected in some other way, the laws of random selection have not been violated, especially when the study is carried out simultaneously at different locations (a multicenter trial.) But do these patients represent the population of patients in the average community? The patients who present for referral may be different from patients at large in several ways, even if they have the same disease as their community counterparts. First, they showed up. This fact alone might indicate that these patients are more astute about their medical care or might have easier access to the medical system. They might be more compliant and might pay more attention to diet and other environmental factors that are not accounted for in the study. They might have more inclusive insurance and be able to afford better health care and all the recommended medications. They might be less sick than those not referred, or more concerned about their health. These could be some of the unaccounted factors that could potentially influence the results of a study.

Somehow, the fact that these patients walk through the referral door makes them different from their community counterparts. We are becoming more aware that the results of major studies from referral centers are not always reproducible to the same extent in the community. It is often necessary to observe the community results of a particular intervention over several years to get an accurate estimate of the effect when used in practice. This process is known as *external validation* as opposed to *internal validation*, which refers to following correct statistical procedure during the study. Refer to Figure 4-3.

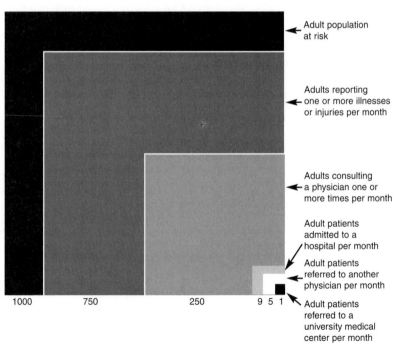

FIGURE 4-3 This illustrates the selectiveness of the referral pattern in health care. The patients referred to a university medical center are only a very small portion of those in the community with the same disease. They may not represent an entirely random sample of the population. (*Redrawn from Figure 1 of White, K., T. Williams, and B. Greenberg. 1961. The ecology of medical care. N Engl J Med, 265:885–892, with permission.*)

KEY POINTS

- It is often impossible to study every member of a population.
- Samples are chosen to represent members of the population at large.
- The law of random sampling states that each member of a population has an equal chance of being chosen for the sample.
- The law of independence states that the selection of one member for the sample does not influence the selection of another.
- If the above laws are followed, each sample of size N has an equal chance of being selected.
- Samples allow you to *estimate* the result you would observe had you studied the entire population.
- Attributes that are observed in a sample are called statistics, whereas the true values in a population are called parameters.
- Because we do not study the entire population, we do not know the true value of the parameter.
- Sample statistics are an estimate of the population parameter.
- Because the statistic is an estimate, it is reported with a range of values on either side known as the confidence interval. If the experiment were repeated multiple times, the confidence interval would fail to include the population parameter about 5% of the time.
- Larger samples result in more accurate estimates of the population parameter. They have narrower confidence intervals.
- Smaller samples may not have enough subjects to detect a true treatment difference if one exists. There is a formula to estimate the minimum number of subjects needed to minimize this type of error.
- The results of studies done in large referral centers are often not exactly reproducible in the community because the sample may not be representative of the population.

REFERENCE

1. Schork, M. A. and Remington, R. D. 2000. *Statistics with applications to the biological and health sciences,* 3rd ed. Upper Saddle River, NJ: Prentice Hall.

REVIEW QUESTIONS

1. Because we cannot study every member of a population, we choose a _____ that represents the population.

2. The sample data result in a sample_____, which is an _____ of the population parameter.

3. If a sample is chosen following the laws of _____ _____ the sample statistic and its confidence interval will very often encompass the population _____ if the experiment were repeated multiple times.

4. In general, larger samples have _____ confidence intervals.

5. Smaller samples are limited in their ability to detect a _____ _____, if one truly exists.

6. Patients participating in studies at large referral centers may not represent the population because the selection process may be _____.

ANSWERS TO REVIEW QUESTIONS

1. sample

2. statistic, estimate

3. random selection, parameter

4. narrower or smaller

5. treatment difference

6. biased or flawed or not random

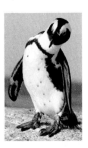

CHAPTER 5

Invariably Variables

Statistics is a tool that helps data produce knowledge rather than confusion.

—David S. Moore and George P. McCabe[1]

If you were to pick up a textbook of statistics, the first chapter would invariably be about variables. It is time to start thinking about populations in terms of their variables and to incorporate this idea into your knowledge base. This lays the foundation for the actual comparison between groups. The concept of a variable is actually quite simple.

- *A variable is any measurable characteristic found in each individual in a population.*

Notice that this definition is very broad. There could be a limitless amount of variables (or measurable characteristics) that could potentially be identified in any population. Not all variables are important to the topic being studied. The investigators choose the variables that are most likely to be useful in determining the end result.

Variables are used to estimate population parameters. A given variable can be measured in each subject from the sample. An example is the variable "age." Every member will have a value associated with age. These values can be used to derive a sample statistic which estimates the population parameter of *average age* or the *standard deviation of age.*

TYPES OF VARIABLES

The variables to be studied are measured in each individual of the sample that has been selected to represent the population. Numerical values are assigned to represent the value of a variable for an individual. Numbers are needed so that calculations can be made, even if the numbers do not directly represent the value of the characteristic. Take gender, for instance. Each subject is either male or female. For statistical purposes, this is often recorded as 0 for male and 1 for female (or vice versa).

Another example is the declared major in a sample of college students. This variable cannot be measured numerically but, for statistical purposes, a 1 can be assigned for Psychology, a 2 for History, a 3 for Biology, and so forth. Note that in these examples the number assigned to the variable does not represent a true numerical value.

These types of variables are called *categorical* variables. Numbers are assigned to the subsets within the category so that a computer can perform calculations to analyze the data. These types of variables have a category key to decipher what the numerical values mean.

Other variables can be easily represented by numbers that directly reflect the value for that individual. These variables are referred to as *quantitative* variables. Yearly income is a good example of this. The number of dollars earned per year by an individual is directly representative of the true value of the characteristic. Another example is number of miles driven on a daily commute to work. The actual number has a real meaning; more miles driven is reflected in a higher numeric value.

You may come across other definitions for different types of variables. For instance, gender can be described as a *binary* or *dichotomous* variable, since there are only two possible values. The answers to questions with a "yes" or "no" answer (such as "Do you own a car?") can also be considered dichotomous variables. It is not important to remember the various ways of describing variables, but you should know that different types of statistical tests are used for analyzing different types of variables.

Inherent in the definition of a variable is the fact that they do indeed *vary*. Different individuals will have different values of a particular variable. In some cases, the value will be only one of two possible choices, as in gender. Other variables will have several limited possibilities, such as college major. When the possible values are limited, the variables are called *discrete*. Variables such as annual income or serum cholesterol level, however, can have a wide variety of responses within a numeric range. These are referred to as *continuous* variables since there is an extensive range of possible values on a continuous scale.

SCALES OF MEASUREMENT

The different types of variables have led to another classification of variables based on the scale of measurement used to determine their value. It is not necessary to memorize these but it is useful to know that they exist. There are four classic scales of measurement:

Nominal scale. This is not really a scale at all; it is a labeling system. Categorical variables such as gender and college major are measured like this. Even though numbers are assigned to the categories, they do not have a true numerical value. They are more like the numbers on football jerseys that designate the different members of a team, without quantitative value.

Ordinal scale. In this scale, a value is given to the variable based on its place along some continuum. The relative place of the variable has some numeric meaning. For instance, we may want to measure the place of the runners in a race as they cross the finish line. First- and second-place runners may wind up being closer together than the second- and third-place runners, but this kind of scale pays attention to *rank* only. Using this scale, the difference between first and second place is the same as between second and third. Quality of life issues are often measured on ordinal scales. Consider a scale that measures overall contentment with regard to medical conditions, with 1 being lowest and 100 being highest. In a population of people who have undergone amputation, a subject who reports a quality of life of 95 has a higher contentment rating than someone who reports 85, who in turn is more content than someone reporting 75. However, in the scale that measures contentment we cannot say that the difference of 10 between the three individuals is equivalent.

Interval scale. This scale is used to measure continuous variables that have legitimate mathematical values. The difference between two consecutive values is consistent along any point of the scale. Many variables can be measured this way. For example, the variable yearly income is used to measure buying power. Someone who makes $60,000 per year has twice as much buying power as someone who makes $30,000 and half as much buying power as those who make $120,000 per year.

Ratio scale. This scale has a true zero point. It is useful for making comparisons between different sets of variables using different scales. The relative distance of the value from zero for one variable can be compared with another. This scale is not used very often in biostatistics.

The *value* of a variable is obviously important. These values are incorporated into the mathematical formulas that eventually produce the answer that is being sought. However, there are many different ways of looking at data and making comparisons. Particular types of variables use distinct statistical tests to draw conclusions. These tests employ different mathematical formulas depending on the type of the gap between consecutive values. Therefore, *it is the type of variable and scale of measurement that determines the legitimate statistical test that is ultimately used to form a conclusion about the data.* In fact, the ability to claim that a difference is "statistically significant" can depend on the scale of measurement and the type of analysis. It is up to the researcher to choose among the alternate methods of treating the data that will result in the most valid conclusion.

Once again, it is not necessary to know the math in order to apply the principles. It is helpful, however, to know that categorical data (such as gender) are treated differently from rank data (such as runners in a race), which are handled differently from continuous data (such as income). Also keep in mind that, for ease of handling, some investigators may treat continuous data like rank data by grouping them. Income is often represented this way. We are all familiar with surveys that ask for a yearly income group instead of actual income (e.g., 0–$20,000, $20,000–$50,000, and so forth). Grouping data consolidates the information and still gives valid conclusions, but a different statistical test may be used during analysis.

The chart in Table 5-1 was recently published in the Seventh Report of the Joint National Committee on the Prevention, Detection, Evaluation and Treatment of High Blood Pressure. This group reviewed the literature on hypertension and recommended guidelines for treating patients. Even though blood pressure is a continuous variable, several ranges of values were demarcated so that categories were created. This is a common way to handle data since it appeals to the human instinct to group and sort. Another example we have seen is the GFR groupings for the level of kidney disease in Figure 2-9 in Chapter 2.

At this point (if you are feeling a little adventurous), turn to Appendix A. This flow diagram shows the different types of statistical tests that are used to analyze data, depending on the type of variables and scale of measurement as well as other factors we have not discussed yet. It can be rather intimidating but it illustrates the steps taken by statisticians as they decide on the appropriate formulas to apply to the data.

TABLE 5-1 Classification and Management of Blood Pressure for Adults Aged 18 Years or Older

BP Classification	Systolic BP, mmHg*		Diastolic BP, mmHg*	Management* Lifestyle Modification	Initial Drug Therapy Without Compelling Indications	Without Compelling Indications
Normal	<120	and	<80	Encourage		
Prehypertension	120–139	or	80–89	Yes	No antihypertensive drug indicated	Drug(s) for the compelling indications[†]
Stage 1 hypertension	140–159	or	90–99	Yes	Thiazide-type diuretics for most; may consider ACE inhibitor, ARB, β-blocker, CCB, or combination	Drug(s) for the compelling indications Other antihypertensive drugs (diuretics, ACE inhibitor, ARB, β-blocker, CCB) as needed
Stage 2 hypertension	>160	or	>100	Yes	2-drug combination for most (usually thiazide-type diuretic and ACE inhibitor or ARB or β-blocker or CCB)[§]	Drug(s) for the compelling indications Other antihypertensive drugs (diuretics, ACE inhibitor, ARB, β-blocker, CCB) as needed

ACE, angiotensin-converting enzyme; ARB, angiotensin receptor blocker; BP, blood pressure; CCB, calcium channel blocker.
*Treatment determined by highest BP category.
[†]Treat patients with chronic kidney disease or diabetes to BP goal of less than 130/80 mmHg.
[§]Combined therapy should be used cautiously in those at risk for orthostatic hypotension.
(From Chobanian AV, Bakris GL, et al., 2003. *JAMA*, 289:29, 2561, with permission.)

Even though the formulas differ, they all produce a p value that is interpreted in the same way. It is not necessary to memorize the appropriate test for each situation. You should still be able to interpret the result no matter what test was used.

A much simpler version of the visual display is shown in Appendix B. Note that the first distinction in the tree depends on the type of variable and scale of measurement. Even though this visual display is not quite as inclusive as the other, it is apparent that different types of data have their own distinct types of statistical tests.

DATA SETS

At first glance, data sets appear to be quite . . .

repetitive	*incessant*	*boring*
monotonous	tedious	tiresome
redundant	mundane	dull . . .

. . . and they are! That is why we have computers do all the work. However, it is good to know how data sets are organized because they are really not as confusing as they seem. A data set is a grid of cells that contain the values of the variables being measured. Along the top are the names of the variables, which form columns. The first column is reserved for the subjects, who are often given a numerical designation. These subject numbers are obviously not included in the final analysis. The rows, which are aligned horizontally, show all the values of the variables for a particular subject. The simplest data set has four cells (two subjects with a measured variable for each). The more complex ones can house millions of cells.

The following sample data set was taken from Moore and McCabe.[1] The investigators were wondering why a particularly large proportion of first-year computer science majors at a large university did not graduate in this major. The data in Table 5-2 were collected on computer science freshmen after three semesters.

TABLE 5-2 Computer Science Freshmen Data Collected after Three Semesters

OBS	GPA	HSM	HSS	HSE	SATM	SATV	SEX
001	3.32	10	10	10	670	600	1
002	2.26	6	8	5	700	640	1
003	2.35	8	6	8	640	530	1
004	2.08	9	10	7	670	600	1
005	3.38	8	9	8	540	580	1

Complete results of the study are reported in Campbell, P. F. and G. P. McCabe, 1984. Predicting the success of freshmen in a computer science major. *Communications of the ACM*, 27, 1108–1113, with permission.

This excerpt includes the first five subjects in a typical data set. Along the top are headings for the variables. The first column is Observation or Subjects (OBS). The numbers 001 to 005 are randomly assigned to individual students; they have no numeric value. GPA is grade point average after three semesters. This could be considered interval data with a range of 0 to 4.0. The variables are continuous since they could take any value within this range.

HSM, HSS, and HSE represent high school scores in math, science, and English, respectively. The scale is 0 to 10, with 10 being an A, 9 being A−, 8 being B+, and so forth. Because the variables have limited values, they could be considered discrete (there is no such value as 9.3, for example). The scale may be considered an interval type if the difference between an A and a B is considered the same as the difference between a B and a C. If the investigators believe that this type of grading scale is universal (an A at one high school equals an A at any of the others), a ratio scale could be considered in the final analysis. SATM and SATV represent testing scores in math and verbal ability. These are continuous variables measured on an interval scale. The last column is gender, which was recorded as 1 for men and 2 for women. This is an example of a discrete, dichotomous variable using a nominal scale.

This limited data set illustrates the different types of variables that can be studied. It is also apparent that even simplistic data can be handled in different ways—all of them arguably correct—depending on the question being asked and the assumptions being made. It is not uncommon for two experienced statisticians to disagree on the finer points of analysis. One way to avoid these conflicts is to decide on the type of statistical tests to be used in a study *before* the data are collected.

Again, it is not necessary to know how the math was done. Just be aware that there are different ways of handling data, which depend on the types of variables and the assumptions being made by the investigators. When you evaluate a study, you may be able to identify some of these assumptions by noting the type of statistical test that was used.

EXPLANATORY AND RESPONSE VARIABLES

When a study is set up to measure the effect of one or more variables on another, there is an assumption that certain variables may have an impact on the result (the dependent variable). Statisticians refer to these contributing variables as *explanatory* variables since they help to explain the outcome. They affect the end result. The dependent variable is called the *response* variable. There is more than just an association among the explanatory variables and the response variable; the presence and quantity of the explanatory variables actually determine the value of the outcome.

For instance, a researcher might want to study the effect of alcohol intake on driver response time. S/he might label blood alcohol level as the explanatory variable. Time lapsed from viewing a red light to putting a foot on a brake pedal could be the response variable. It seems likely that an increased value of the blood alcohol level will be associated with longer response times. There is more than just an association between the two variables here; one has an effect on the other.

The above scenario might suggest that the presence of one variable *causes* the effect on the other. However, proving causality is a little more intricate than just an observation that a given variable has an effect on the response. Multiple prospective studies with concurring results need to be done before the scientific community will accept a cause-and-effect relationship between two variables. One of the stronger arguments that support a cause-and-effect relationship is if the effect disappears when the explanatory variable is removed.

KEY POINTS

- A variable is any measurable characteristic found in each individual in a population.
- Categorical variables are assigned numbers that represent categories. The numbers have no numerical value.
- Quantitative variables have a number that represents a value.
- There are four classic scales of measurement that variables fall into: Nominal, Ordinal, Interval, and Ratio. (NOIR. French, anyone?)
- The type of variable and scale of measurement are used to determine the appropriate statistical test to answer the research question.
- It is possible that a continuous variable can be grouped so that a different scale of measurement is used, depending on the assumptions made by the investigators who decide on the most valid way to handle the data.
- Data sets are organized into cells that contain values of the variables under investigation.
- The explanatory variable has an effect on the response variable but does not necessarily prove causation.

REFERENCE

1. Moore, D. S. and G. P. McCabe. 1999. *Introduction to the practice of statistics,* 3rd ed. New York: W. H. Freeman and Co.

REVIEW QUESTIONS

1. A variable is a measurable characteristic with _____ possible values.

2. _____ variables are assigned a number even though they have no numeric value.

3. _____ of measurement and _____ of variable determine the statistical test that is used.

4. In the graph of income versus schooling (Figure 2-8 in Chapter 2), _____ is the response variable since _____ helps to explain level of income.

5. In the graph of kidney failure (Figure 2-9 in Chapter 2), _____ is the response variable since _____.

6. The results of a study may vary if a variable is measured on a different scale. It is up to the _____ and _____ to determine the most valid scale of measurement and statistical test.

ANSWERS TO REVIEW QUESTIONS

1. two or more (depending on the type of variable)
2. Categorical
3. Scale, type
4. yearly income, years of schooling
5. serum creatinine, kidney function has an effect on creatinine levels
6. investigators, statisticians

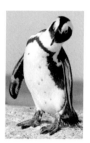

CHAPTER 6

Outcomes

Health is "*a state of complete physical, mental and social well-being and not merely the absence of disease or infirmity.*"

—*World Health Organization*

We have declared that the mission of the health care professional is to help people live longer and feel better by identifying pathways that contribute to those benefits. Research identifies these pathways by observing what happens over time to a sample that is divided into groups and exposed to different interventions. If one group has a measurable advantage over the other in the "live longer/feel better" category, we can recommend this pathway to an individual who belongs to the population that sample represents.

This chapter is devoted to a certain type of variable that has the noble distinction of representing our mission. It attempts to capture the live longer/feel better condition in people. This unique variable is referred to as the *outcome variable*. Outcome variables measure live longer/feel better by contributing to at least one of these two categories.

QUALITY-ADJUSTED LIFE-YEARS (QUALY)

"Live longer" is fairly easy to measure. Obviously, it can be measured in terms of life-years. In other words, we can say that one group as a whole does better if more people are alive at the end of the study. Live-longer measurements are not complicated; they are essentially mortality rates. The benefit from living longer is readily apparent and openly endorsed in most conditions.

It is important, however, to consider the quality of those life-years that are bestowed upon individuals. It is not always beneficial to extend life if each day is a burden. The enjoyment factor is an important part of an individual's overall satisfaction. There has been a recent surge of interest in methods used to quantify the quality of life (QOL). This outcome is obviously more difficult to measure than life-years since it tends to be subjective and variable among individuals with the same restrictions. In spite of the inherent limitations of this type of research, gallant advances using sophisticated techniques are being made in this arena in an attempt to quantify the so-called well-being factor.

Most QOL measurements are done by questionnaire. The surveys are completed by individuals who have the disease being studied, or by caregivers when the subject is unable to respond. These instruments often use Likert scales to measure graded responses (e.g., poor, fair, good, very good, excellent). They undergo rigorous testing for validity and reliability before they are released for use. *Validity* addresses the question of whether an instrument measures what is intended. Most methods to check for validity employ another external measure to see how the methods correlate. *Reliability* is a reflection of reproducibility. A reliable instrument will show some variability but will demonstrate consistency over time.

Some surveys cover generic QOL issues, such as the Short Form Health Status Questionnaire, known as the SF-36^R. This instrument poses 36 questions that cover multiple health-related categories (also known as domains). These attempt to measure physical, emotional, social, and cognitive levels of functioning. They can therefore be used in various situations to assess general functional status and overall well-being. There are several versions of this type of questionnaire. Figure 6-1 shows a breakdown of the types of domains that are captured in one of these instruments.

Figure 6-2 shows the results when a cross section of patients with varying types of diseases were asked to evaluate their QOL using a generic measure known as the Sickness Impact Profile score. These are descriptive data that compare different disease states in terms of perceived overall well-being, although the results were not adjusted for age or other factors and the disease states shown are by no means all-inclusive. The longer bars represent poorer QOL perception.

Most of the results are predictable. As expected, patients with chronic disease states causing uncontrollable pain reported poorer QOL in general. Those who reported the worst QOL in this study had a progressive degenerative neurological disorder called amyotrophic lateral sclerosis (ALS, or Lou Gehrig's disease), which causes lack of strength and motor control but (perhaps regrettably) does not affect intellectual function. It is conceivable that these unfortunate individuals might be compelled to engage a professional to assist in life-ending measures.

On the other hand, a rather surprising result shows that those who have suffered cardiac arrest report an incredibly good quality of life! These folks often have no permanent impairment once the event is reversed, and they may reflect upon their good fortune. Perhaps those who have seen the light at the end of the tunnel are more appreciative of the fact that they are alive, and their other maladies become unimportant by comparison.

In addition to general QOL measures, other instruments focus on disease-specific issues related to QOL. These are more applicable in chronic, prevalent diseases and can also be used to make comparisons over time within the same sample. For instance, surveys have been developed to measure the QOL experienced by patients with congestive heart failure (CHF.) The often-quoted New York Heart Association classification[1] is a simple instrument that assesses the level of symptoms experienced by the individual, using Class I (asymptomatic during normal activities) through Class IV (symptoms occur at rest.) Physicians use this classification to monitor the success of treatment in the individual patient. It is also applied to groups of CHF patients to assess the efficacy of large-scale programs and interventions.

Concurrent physical and psychological conditions that contribute to an individual's outlook can affect the validity of a QOL measurement. For instance, a person with chronic pain from an orthopedic condition may also suffer from depression, which would decrease his or her QOL. It can be quite challenging to tease

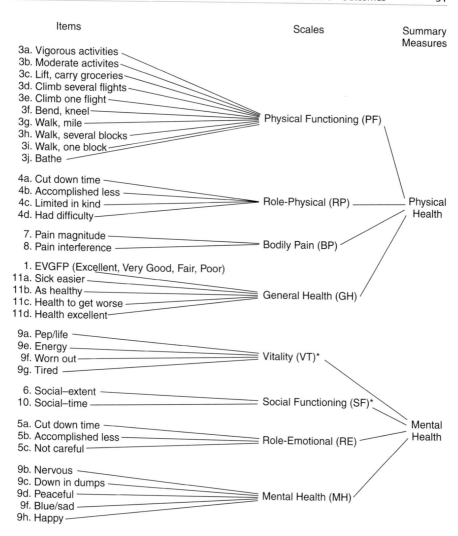

Items   Scales   Summary Measures

3a. Vigorous activities
3b. Moderate activites
3c. Lift, carry groceries
3d. Climb several flights
3e. Climb one flight
3f. Bend, kneel
3g. Walk, mile
3h. Walk, several blocks
3i. Walk, one block
3j. Bathe

Physical Functioning (PF)

4a. Cut down time
4b. Accomplished less
4c. Limited in kind
4d. Had difficulty

Role-Physical (RP)

7. Pain magnitude
8. Pain interference

Bodily Pain (BP)

1. EVGFP (Excellent, Very Good, Fair, Poor)
11a. Sick easier
11b. As healthy
11c. Health to get worse
11d. Health excellent

General Health (GH)

Physical Health

9a. Pep/life
9e. Energy
9f. Worn out
9g. Tired

Vitality (VT)*

6. Social–extent
10. Social–time

Social Functioning (SF)*

5a. Cut down time
5b. Accomplished less
5c. Not careful

Role-Emotional (RE)

Mental Health

9b. Nervous
9c. Down in dumps
9d. Peaceful
9f. Blue/sad
9h. Happy

Mental Health (MH)

* Significant correlation with other summary measure.

FIGURE 6-1 The SF-36ᴿ is a simple questionnaire that attempts to capture overall well-being.

out such interdependent factors. If the investigators want to exclude people with clinical depression from their sample, they would screen for depression and exclude those subjects.

Unlike life-years, QOL measures also attempt to capture the unwelcome side effects of a treatment, which can range from a bothersome rash to a life-threatening complication such as bone marrow failure. If a side effect of treatment results in a hospital admission, QOL measures can reflect this adverse event even though the subject's life may be prolonged overall. Most studies will mention the severity and incidence of adverse

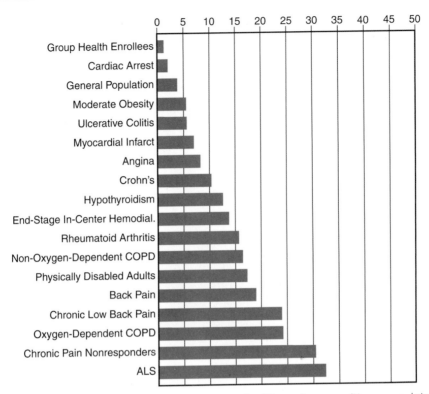

FIGURE 6-2 Overall Sickness Impact Profile (SIP) scores for different disease conditions or population groups. Higher scores reflect poorer quality of life (QOL). (*Patrick D. L. and R. A. Deyo, 1989. Generic and disease: specific measures in assessing health status and quality of life.* Medical Care, *27(suppl):3, 5220.*)

effects even when QOL is not measured. It is assumed that these complications have a negative impact on overall QOL.

A combination of life-years and QOL is captured in the outcome measure known as quality-adjusted life-years (QUALY). This measures not only longevity but also the contentment that is experienced each year. In theory, QUALY fully captures the response to a given treatment and represents live longer/feel better for a period of a year.

- *Quality-adjusted life-years (QUALY) is the quintessential outcome measure.*

In practice, however, QOL is difficult to measure. In many instances, the data are just not available to incorporate into the statistical analysis. In these cases, only mortality rates are used to track outcomes. There is a common assumption that it is better to be alive than dead. (I think most of us would agree!) This leap is justified in conditions that have negligible impact on overall QOL, or if a person's discomfort is limited to a relatively short period of time. However, when you see a study that does not address QOL and you think one of the treatment arms may have a significantly negative impact on a patient's well-being, be sure to incorporate that into your evaluation of the authors' final recommendation.

THE POWER OF PREVENTION

The restoration of QUALYs can be best appreciated when an individual undergoes a life-saving procedure. For example, the successful surgical repair of an acutely ruptured aorta saves the victim from certain death in a dramatic intervention. The QUALYs bestowed during this emergent procedure can be appreciated by anyone who is even remotely aware of the gravity of this particular condition.

However, do not underestimate the power of *prevention* in bestowing QUALYs. For instance, the prevention of vascular disease by appropriate lifestyle habits is a very cost-effective way to provide QUALYs. The patient with mild hypertension who smokes heavily would be much better off giving up the nicotine sticks rather than starting a medication for the minimal elevation in blood pressure. It behooves us as health care providers to emphasize to our patients the importance of healthy habits.

The beneficial effect of prevention is even more potent when considering certain childhood diseases. The humble immunization has provided for an immense number of additional QUALYs—more than any invasive intervention could ever hope to parallel. A simple shot or a squirt of liquid in the nose, when given to the multitude, has a potential beneficial effect on not just the individual but on the population as well. Not everyone would have gotten the disease but, by immunizing everyone, we prevent the disease from afflicting anyone. Since most of these diseases occur in childhood, the number of QUALYs imparted to those individuals who would have otherwise been robbed of their adult life (or, as in the case of polio survivors, forced to live with a handicap) is tremendous.

The difference between a dramatic intervention that saves an individual, versus preventing a disease in the community and thus saving many lives, is that the benefit in the prevention scenario is often not fully appreciated. We tend to notice when an individual who is hovering at death's door is miraculously pulled back. We are less likely to be aware of the impact of prevention on averting bad outcomes. Prevention is a very powerful tool in providing additional QUALYs to large groups of people.

SURROGATE OUTCOME VARIABLES

You will undoubtedly encounter many clinical studies that do not use the ideal outcome variable, QUALY. If all studies waited patiently to measure mortality rates in their subjects before being published, *we* would likely be dead before the results were available! If an investigator knows that certain other outcomes are associated with higher mortality rates or decreased QOL, s/he might substitute these proxy variables for QUALY. It is a commonly accepted practice to use surrogate markers that indirectly reflect QUALYs, especially when a direct QUALY measurement cannot be reasonably obtained and the surrogate is relatively easy to measure. The surrogate marker that is substituted should have a direct correlation with the outcome it represents. It is more difficult, however, to accurately quantify the impact of an intervention on QUALY when a surrogate marker is substituted.

An example of this application is seen in studies that use carotid wall thickness as a marker of atherosclerosis. The thickness of the inner and middle portions of blood vessel walls can easily be measured using a noninvasive ultrasound technique. Since this is associated with the progression of coronary artery disease, it has been used as an index to follow the evolution of subclinical cardiovascular disease. It has also been used as a surrogate measure of cardiovascular disease outcomes.[2]

EVENT-FREE SURVIVAL

Investigators who oversee clinical studies are concerned with minimizing the chance of a bad outcome in a population. The better pathway will have more healthy survivors at the end of the study. Another outcome measure often encountered in the literature is *event-free survival*, which approximates QUALY. This outcome tracks the major adverse events that decrease QUALY but does not weight them according to their individual effect on QUALY. Anyone who avoids a major adverse outcome, such as heart attack, stroke, or death, is designated as an event-free survivor when comparisons are made between the pathways at the end of the study. This type of outcome accounts for the major conditions that affect QUALY but does not consider smaller decreases in QUALY, such as those that might be related to medication side effects.

COMPOSITE OUTCOMES

It is also very common to see studies that track the opposite of QUALYs—the adverse events and deaths that occur in the groups. These are sometimes referred to as *hazards*. It is not always necessary to focus on a solitary condition responsible for a bad outcome, especially when any of several related diseases could have been the culprit.

For instance, vascular disease affects the blood vessels in many organs. As vascular disease progresses, a person is at increasing risk of heart attack or stroke. Both of these can result in death or permanent disability. It does not matter anatomically where the deleterious event occurs; the individual still suffers the bad outcome. When the potential outcomes are linked, the outcome variable can be combined to include several possibilities. The subjects are then observed to see whether *any* of the outcomes happen. This is referred to as a *composite outcome*.

The various outcomes are each identified as a deleterious event, so the difference in risk between the two groups becomes evident sooner than if a solitary event was the primary endpoint. The additive rule of probability is used. For instance (and this is purely speculative), if in one arm of a study the risk of stroke was observed to be 2% per year and the risk of heart attack was 3% per year, the risk of heart attack *or* stroke was 5% per year, or 5 out of 100 (assuming no subject gets both).

Composite outcomes are not concurrent in an individual. If we were tracking the risk of heart attack *and* stroke, we would use the multiplicative rule which multiplies individual risks. In the above example, the risk of having both would be about 0.06% per year, or 6 out of 10,000. (This argument assumes that these disease entities are independent and not linked, but in fact they most likely are. This would change the formula somewhat.)

If we tracked concurrent outcomes, we would have to wait an extremely long time before any advantage could be appreciated in one group over the other, since the incidence of the concurrent outcome is low to begin with. Combining outcomes in this additive way allows a difference in risk to be appreciated much sooner. Many published studies use the word *and* when defining their combined outcomes, when in actuality the more appropriate word is *or*. Combining outcomes has the main advantage of shortening the length of time necessary to observe the subjects. The answer to the question of which pathway has the greater advantage will be apparent sooner if several linked adverse effects are tracked simultaneously.

The HOPE trial in 2000[3] used a composite outcome of myocardial infarction, stroke, *or* death from cardiovascular disease when studying the effect of ramipril on a population of people at risk for vascular events over an average of 5 years. Myocardial infarction and stroke can both have a severe impact on QOL. This was combined with mortality from heart disease as the major outcome variable, or *primary endpoint*. Each outcome can also be analyzed separately. In this study, ramipril had a beneficial effect in reducing the rate of the combined outcome and the individual outcomes as well.

KEY POINTS

- The outcome variable is the measurement of live longer/feel better at the end of the study.
- "Live longer" is measured in mortality.
- "Feel better" is measured in quality of life.
- Combining these outcome measures results in Quality-Adjusted Life Years (QUALY), the quintessential outcome measure.
- Surrogate measures can be substituted as outcome measures if they correlate with "live longer" or "feel better," but the measurable effect may be more difficult to quantify than if a true QUALY measure was used.
- Composite outcomes combine multiple adverse events into one measurement.
- Using composite outcomes can decrease the time needed to observe a treatment difference between the groups.
- Prevention can be a very effective way to bestow additional QUALYs, although its impact may not be readily apparent.

REFERENCES

1. www.hcoa.org/hcoacme/chf.cme/chf 00070.htm, 2005.
2. O'Leary, D. H. et al. 2002. Intima-media thickness: A tool for atherosclerosis imaging and event prediction. *Am J Cardiol*, 90(suppl), 18L–21L.
3. The HOPE Study Investigators. 2000. Effect of an angiotensin-converting enzyme inhibitor, ramipril, on cardiovascular events in high-risk patients. *New Engl J Med*, 342:3, 145.

REVIEW QUESTIONS

1. The mission of health care professionals is to improve the human condition by helping people to _____ _____ and _____ _____.

2. "Live longer" is measured as _____.

3. "Feel better" is measured as _____ ___ _____.

4. _____ is an attempt to capture these combined outcome measures.

5. _____ is an effective way to bestow QUALYs.

6. An effective prevention or treatment measure decreases the _____ to a population of a bad outcome over time.

7. _____ outcomes can help to shorten the length of a study.

ANSWERS TO REVIEW QUESTIONS

1. live longer, feel better

2. mortality

3. quality of life

4. Quality-adjusted life years or QUALY

5. Prevention

6. risk

7. Combined, composite

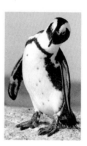

CHAPTER 7

Probability

The revolutionary idea that defines the boundary between modern times and the past is the mastery of risk: the notion that the future is more than a whim of the gods and that men and women are not passive before nature.

—*Peter L. Bernstein*[1]

The science of inferential statistics did not develop overnight. It evolved over hundreds of years from basic mathematical principles into a discipline that uses observations to predict the future. The probability theories upon which inferential statistics is built were revealed sequentially through a diligent process that reflects several centuries of intellectual curiosity and pursuit.

THE HISTORY OF PROBABILITY THEORY

Statistics is a relatively recent product of the last few centuries. The earliest counting systems were able to keep track of large numbers of items, but did not allow for the abstract idea of "none" or for negative numbers. The modern arithmetic that we use today had its humble origin about 1500 years ago, when the Hindus developed a numbering system that incorporated the concept of zero. This notion allowed for the development of a more standard approach to counting in which a limited number of digits (0 through 9) could be placed side-by-side, and their relative value depended on the column (1s, 10s, 100s, etc.) they occupied. Now there was no limit on the value that a number could express.

The Arabs adopted the new system when they traveled throughout India, and developed it further. In the ninth century an Arabic mathematician named Al-Khowarizmi wrote one of the earliest mathematical works on simple algebraic equations. His name ultimately evolved into the word *algorithm*, which means "rules for computing." Another of his works, *Hisab al-jabr w' almuqabalah*, which means "science of transposition and cancellation," gives us the word for *algebra* (*al-jabr*). The new numbers were met with some resistance in Western Europe, but over the next few centuries they were eventually adopted as a logical way of expressing values and solving equations. This novel system allowed for the development of probability theory, which is based on equations that enable us to quantify risk.

Humans like the comfort of predictable outcomes, but we live in an imperfect world. We strive to make failure-free devices, but any equipment we produce will have a failure rate. We cannot say with confidence that a bad event will not happen when we travel. We also cannot guarantee that a recommended treatment will work. We have no choice but to accept some uncertainty about the future. However, guided by the laws of probability, we can make informed choices that allow us to maximize the chance of a good outcome.

The radical concept that humans could predict outcomes is relatively new. Until the past few centuries, people believed that future events were controlled by an omnipotent deity. They were powerless to mold their destiny. Without the framework of the science of logic, they relied on the alluring predictions of mystics and soothsayers. As laws of physics were discovered during the Middle Ages, people began to realize that there was some order to the events of the heavens and the physical world. Only then did the aura of mysticism surrounding secular events began to dissolve.

People have always been intrigued by games of chance. Evidence of gambling has been found on Egyptian paintings that date back as early as 3500 B.C., and accounts of this pastime have been recorded throughout history in all societies and economic classes. As people began to appreciate that their world responded to the laws of physics, they also discovered that certain games had outcomes which could be predicted by mathematical formulas. The desire to predict these outcomes led to an interest in the "science of choice."

Several great works were written during the Renaissance on the topic of chance. One of the most notable was a treatise by a sixteenth-century Italian physician named Girolamo Cardano. He was an avid gambler who developed the algebraic formulas to calculate the expected outcomes when throwing dice. These formulas are used today by casino owners to ensure that they have the advantage in the long run and do not lose money.

The outcomes in games of chance (such as dice) can be calculated mathematically because the chance of each occurrence is known. In a fair game of dice, we know the probability of getting a sum of 7 when two dice are rolled. There are six combinations that could produce a 7 out of a total of 36 possible combinations. The probability formulas allow us to calculate the frequency at which we can expect to roll a 7 when we throw the dice more than once. An analogous situation is the flip of a coin. We know the probability of getting heads is 50% but, using the binomial formulas, we can also calculate the chances of getting heads one-quarter of the time over multiple coin flips.

A century before Cardano's formulas were presented, an Italian monk named Luca Pacioli had posed the question of how the stakes should be divided in an unfinished game when one of the players is ahead. This riddle remained unsolved for two centuries, until 1654, when the famous French mathematicians Pascal and Fermat were able to solve the puzzle by using formulas to predict what would most likely happen if the game kept going.

Predicting chance occurrences in events such as coin flips and rolls of the dice led to more hypothetical inquiries. Is there a way to predict events in which the probability of a particular outcome is unknown? Jacob Bernoulli was a mathematician who was intrigued by the idea of applying probability theory to these abstract situations. In 1713 his essay *Ars Conjectandi* (*The Art of Conjecture*) was published; it suggested that sample data could be used to calculate unknown probabilities. Several years later a minister named Thomas Bayes published a paper that distinguished him as one of the prominent statisticians. In *An Essay Towards Solving a Problem in the Doctrine of Chances*, he presented a system that allowed for the revision of predictions by incorporating new observations. These were some of the more notable contributions that molded probability theory, which allows us to quantify risk.

THE MODERN CONCEPT OF RISK

These discoveries had phenomenal consequences that ultimately led to the development of modern society. People are willing to take a risk if they know the chance of the desired result. No one takes a risk in an entirely futile situation, but being able to calculate the possibility of the desired outcome can justify taking a chance on something with a less than 100% guarantee. The practice of modern medicine has no guarantees. There is a risk involved with every treatment, but being able to predict the risk can justify the path that is chosen. Inferential statistics, with its roots in probability theory, allows us to calculate that risk. The innate human interest in games of chance has led to extraordinary discoveries about the science of predictability. Although the concepts of probability theory seem relatively simple, it took several centuries to unveil them. We stand on the shoulders of mathematical giants such as Pascal and Fermat when we use modern probability calculations to interpret the results of studies that guide us in our daily medical decisions.

The modern application of inferential statistics has continued to develop during the past century. Many recent contributions have resulted in the refinement of a process that now defines standard statistical procedure. R. A. Fisher was an English geneticist who lived during the first half of the twentieth century and worked with agricultural experiments. He is credited with the introduction of randomization into experimental design and the advancement of statistical methods through significance testing. He also introduced the idea of hypothesis testing. The famous statisticians Jerzy Neyman and Egon Pearson explored this idea in more detail around the 1930s. They promoted a hypothesis testing theory based on a decision-making model that applied what are called the null and alternative hypotheses. The ultimate product that evolved is actually a hybrid of ideas that have led us into the era of modern statistical theory.

These developments represent just a few of the recent contributions that have had a significant impact on the evolution of statistical analysis. This science continues to progress even now, as new mathematical formulas are being developed to interpret different types of data and philosophical arguments are made in favor of alternative methodology and interpretation of results.

QUANTIFYING CHANCE OCCURRENCES

Inferential statistics is based on the probability of a certain outcome happening by chance. In probability theory, the word *outcome* refers to the result observed. It does not necessarily reflect quality-adjusted life-years (QUALY) like the outcome variable we see in clinical trials. It is simply the result of an event. The range of probabilities varies between 0 (no probability of the event happening) and 1 (the outcome will always happen.) It is rare to find circumstances in nature where the probability of occurrence is equal to 0 or 1. If that were the case, there would be no need to apply probability theory. All events that are studied in medicine have a probability of occurrence between 0 and 1. This is expressed as a decimal, such as 0.35. The simplest, most informative interpretation of probability converts these values to percentages to express the chance of something happening. An outcome with a probability of 0.35 is said to have a 35% chance of occurrence. On average, it will happen 35 times out of 100 opportunities. It follows that an outcome with 100% probability means there is no possibility that the outcome will not happen (but this never happens!).

A *p* value is really a probability that a given outcome could occur by chance. It is usually expressed as a decimal, such as 0.07. A *p* value, when multiplied by 100, is a percentage. In the above example, the *p* value of 0.07 means that there is a 7% probability that the observed outcome could happen by chance alone. (This is based on an underlying assumption that certain conditions have been met, which we will look into later.) Another way of stating this is: If the study were repeated hundreds of times under the same circumstances, using members of the same population, an average of only seven of these studies out of 100 would give the result we observe based on chance alone. The reason why each study does not give identical results in these situations is because different samples are used, which results in different estimates of the parameter. We will discuss this concept again but, for now, just realize that the *p* value represents a probability, which can be expressed as a percentage.

EVENTS AND OCCURRENCE

When I was a student of biostatistics studying the laws of probability, I came to realize a very sobering concept that deserves emphasis:

- *If something can happen, it will.*

If it is at all possible for an event to occur, no matter how miniscule the chance, it will eventually happen. We may not have seen it yet and may not see it in our lifetime, but it is a mathematical certainty that if the conditions for the event are in place, and given enough chances, it will occur. It may take hundreds of years but it is guaranteed to happen.

The challenge, of course, is knowing in advance that something *can* happen. If it has never been observed, we can only surmise that it is possible if logic tells us so. In cases of rare events, we depend on the experience of others who report them, but we must consider the reliability of the source. Still other events may not have been recognized for what they were, and may have been misreported or overlooked entirely.[2] It is not always apparent that a particular event can occur and, unfortunately, in some circumstances this event can have disastrous consequences.

For instance, it is possible for a distracted factory employee working at a stamping press to slip his hand into the press and suffer an amputation. We know this because it was observed on a rare occasion. Because it can happen, it did. This has led to increased awareness and mandatory educational efforts, but can only be fully prevented if it *cannot* happen. That is why mechanical safeguards were invented and should be enforced. If it is at all possible for a nurse to mistake a solution of potassium chloride for another drug and inject it into a patient, causing a cardiac arrest, it will happen. It may not happen at every institution, but for multiple sites participating in repeated events in which it could happen, someone's number will eventually come up. That is why potassium chloride should not be easily available in an injectable form.

Any of us who work in a health care field should harbor a healthy respect for this particular law of probability. Morbidity and mortality conferences are helpful in hindsight, but making it impossible for an event to occur *before* it happens is the only way to ensure that it *will not* happen. (If something *cannot* happen, it *will not.*) Try to predict the worst possible adverse events that could result from an action and estimate the probability of their occurrence. If a particularly dire event can be prevented, find the easiest way to do this. There are many situations where all adverse events just simply cannot be eliminated; there is risk involved with any intervention. There is also no substitute for good judgment and careful attention to details. But human error does occur, and it behooves us to try to avoid the scenario that invites it rather than blaming the individual. If there is a good way to reduce or erase risk without undue effort, it should be pursued.

KEY POINTS

- The science of biostatistics evolved over many centuries.
- The development of probability theory was driven by interest in gambling and games of chance.
- The quantification of risk allows us to take chances in uncertain circumstances.
- Modern statistical processes are the result of multiple contributions from notable scientists who applied probability theory to hypothesis testing.
- The *p* value is the probability of a chance occurrence.
- If something can happen, it will.

REFERENCES

1. Bernstein, P. L. 1988. *Against the gods: The remarkable story of risk.* New York: John Wiley & Sons, Inc. All references to historical data are from this work.
2. Dr. Bob Wolfe, personal communication, August, 2005.

REVIEW QUESTIONS

1. The probability of certain events can be predicted using mathematical _____.

2. If we know the probability of the occurrence of an event, when the outcomes are known (such as when lottery numbers are drawn) we can calculate the _____ of hitting all the numbers.

3. Even though we may feel an intuition to play certain numbers, we are just as likely to win if we play another set of _____.

4. In the case where the probability of an event is less certain, we base our predictions on prior _____.

5. We can refine the process of quantifying risk by incorporating _____ that affect the outcome.

6. If we wanted to predict the likelihood of getting into a car accident, we could base our overall risk on prior data. If we also considered the time of day, the age of the driver, and

the weather conditions, we could refine the _____ using the methods of Bayes based on observations when these factors were considered.

7. A p value of < 0.01 means that the probability of this event happening by chance alone is less than _____.

ANSWERS TO REVIEW QUESTIONS

1. formulas

2. chance, likelihood, probability

3. numbers

4. observations

5. factors, variables

6. risk, prediction

7. 1 out of 100, 1%

CHAPTER 8

Distributions

A picture is worth a thousand words.

—Anonymous

The numbers in a data set represent values of certain characteristics. Every member of the population will have a value associated with that characteristic, and they will not all be the same value. However, the values often tend to cluster. For instance, in a population of 30-year-olds, the values for systolic blood pressure will vary but they will tend to cluster around 120 mmHg. This is the nature of biologic data. Variables are not uniformly the same but they do tend to congregate around a common value.

When we go on a vacation to a distant location, we want to be able to describe the experience to our friends. We remember the topography of the area, what the temperature was like, and the inhabitants. We take pictures to record different details such as the various plants and flowers, the relief of the land, and the way the native people look. It is much easier for our friends to get an idea of the type of place it is by looking at photos rather than listening to a verbal description.

Just as a collection of photos contains a lot of information about a place, a data set from a sample contains a lot of information about a population. However, it is difficult to see the way a characteristic is distributed by looking at a list of numbers. It is much easier to get a feel for the spread of the individual characteristics by transforming the data into pictures by creating graphs.

In the vacation metaphor, different types of photos are best-suited for representing a given characteristic about the place. For instance, close-ups of faces are more suitable for showing the features of the individuals, whereas wide-angle shots are better at capturing the geography of the area. In the same way, different types of graphs can be used to best represent the spread of the values of a characteristic in a sample. The graph illustrates the pattern of variability, which is known as the variable's *distribution*.

- *A distribution is the pattern observed in a collection of values for a variable.*

There are several ways to demonstrate the pattern of a variable, depending on the type of variable, its scale of measurement, and the range of values. The following examples include the more common types of distributions and illustrate how the pattern of spread can be appreciated by a pictorial display. As we will see, distributions are an important link in the inference process between the data and the conclusion.

TYPES OF DISTRIBUTIONS

When we discussed the types of variables in Chapter 5, we stated that categorical variables may be assigned a number but the number represents a category rather than a true value. Table 8-1 is a data set that contains information on the marital status (a categorical variable) for all Americans age 18 or over. In this example the categories of marital status are listed instead of being assigned a number. The same data are displayed in a different format in Figure 8-1.

Another way to illustrate the distribution of these variables is with a bar graph, as in Figure 8-2. The height of the bar allows easy comparison among the different values of the characteristic. Keep in mind that the ordinate (*y*-axis) represents the frequency of the value. The higher the bar, the more variables in the data set that have that value. This format is known as a *histogram*.

- *A histogram is a type of bar graph in which the height of the bar represents the relative frequency of the observed value in the data set.*

Variables that use an ordinate system can also be displayed in the bar graph, as in Figure 8-3. Recall that these variables have numerical values that indicate their relative place within the group and that the mathematical differences between the numerical values are not consistent. The observed value for the variable has been replaced by a numerical rank, from lowest to highest. It is easy to see if and where the values tend to cluster.

Recall that interval variables have values that represent a continuous scale. These can be displayed most effectively as a graph that actually uses the interval scale as its abscissa (*x*-axis.) The values increase along the *x*-axis in a continuous fashion. Just as with the bar graph, the height of the curve represents the frequency with which we observe that value. This type of graph is called a *frequency distribution*. This particular type of graphic representation is a crucial component of inferential statistics. We will use this type of graph to plot probabilities, which are the basis of inferential statistics.

- *A frequency distribution is a graph that plots the value of a variable against the frequency of occurrence.*

A histogram is a type of frequency distribution. The height of the individual bars represent the relative frequency at which each value occurs. When the bars are placed

---

TABLE 8-1 Count and Percent of Marital Status of Americans Age 18 and Over

Marital Status	Count (millions)	Percent
Never married	43.9	22.9
Married	116.7	60.9
Widowed	13.4	7.0
Divorced	17.6	9.2

Data from Moore, D. S. and G. P. McCabe. 1999. *Introduction to the practice of statistics*, 3rd ed. New York: W. H. Freeman and Co., p. 6.

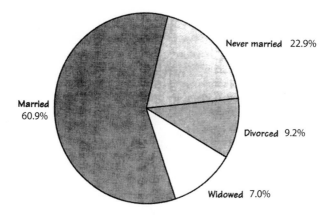

FIGURE 8-1 Pie chart of the same data as in Table 8-1. The human eye immediately compares the area contained within the different slices. The categories need to be mutually exclusive unless there is a slice devoted to a combination of the categories. *(From Moore, D. S. and G. P. McCabe. 1999. Introduction to the practice of statistics, 3rd ed. New York: W. H. Freeman and Co., p. 7, with permission.)*

close together, a pattern emerges. We see in Figure 8-4 that as the values along the abscissa are divided into smaller units, the height of the bars can be connected to form a smooth line.

A *stem and leaf plot* (also called *stemplot*) is a creative way of displaying not only the relative frequency of a value, but the individual values as well. It allows a side-by-side comparison of the distributions of a variable in two groups. This type of plot takes raw data and arranges them into a continuum based on the relative value of each measurement (lowest to highest). The stem plots out what are called the

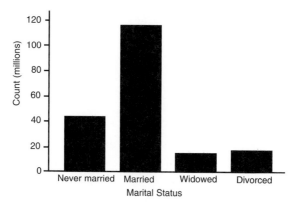

FIGURE 8-2 Bar graph of the marital status of U.S. adults. *(From Moore, D. S. and G. P. McCabe. 1999. Introduction to the practice of statistics, 3rd ed. New York: W. H. Freeman and Co., p. 6, with permission.)*

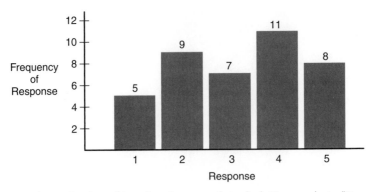

FIGURE 8-3 The results of a poll in a shopping center that asked 40 respondents: "Do you agree with the mayor's position on downtown development?" 1, strongly disagree; 2, disagree; 3, neither agree nor disagree; 4, agree; 5, strongly agree.

leading digits—the higher numbers that encompass many of the values, such as the 100s or 10s. The 1s are plotted individually next to their stem to form the leaves. In Table 8-2, a comparison was made between students who attend class regularly versus those who do not. The total points for each individual in a psychology course are plotted on a stem and leaf diagram. On the right are the regular attendees and on the left are the truants.

The stem is the center of the graph. The first stem of 18 actually represents 180. The leaves represent the 1s. The first entry off to the left side is 8. When tacked on to the stem of 18, it represents a single entry of 188—the lowest total points anyone earned. This person happened to be in the truant group. There are two individuals who earned 195 points. These are plotted next to each other. You can see that they were both in the truant group. The lowest number of points in the attendee group was 241 points; the highest was 328, which was the highest overall.

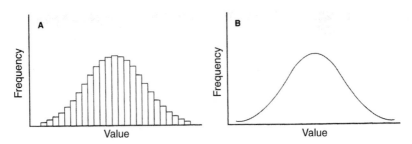

FIGURE 8-4 Example of a frequency distribution. The relative frequency of each value takes on a pattern of symmetry, with the most frequent value in the center of the graph. This pattern of distribution is often observed in nature. *(From Jekel, J. et al. 2001. Epidemiology, biostatistics, and preventive medicine, 2nd ed. Philadelphia: Saunders, p. 142.)*

TABLE 8-2 Psychology Class Earned Points

Missed Class Often	Stem	Attended Regularly
8	18	
5 5	19	
	20	
	21	
8 5	22	
9 7 3 2	23	
0	24	1 3 6 9
6 6 6 0	25	0 2 4 4 5 6
8 4 4 1	26	1 2 3 4 4 4 5 7 7
7 4 4 0 0	27	0 1 2 3 6 6 7 8 8
	28	0 1 2 4 8 8
	29	0 1 1 2 3 4 6 6 7 8
8	30	
	31	0
	32	0 1 8

Code |25| 6 = 256

Total number of points earned in a psychology class by those who attended class regularly versus those who did not.
Data from Howell, D. C. 1999. *Fundamental statistics for the behavioral sciences*, 4th ed. Pacific Grove, CA: Duxbury Press, p. 37.

When you scan this pictograph, several points become immediately apparent. The no-shows got fewer points overall than did the more conscientious students. Looking at the tendency to cluster, the overall average points for the slackers are lower. Also, the spread of points in the truant group is splayed wider than that of the attendees. The points range from the worst to the fifth-highest. Some truant students were able to score pretty well; perhaps they had an alternative method of learning. Only one was able to do very well, however. It obviously helps to go to class, unless you are one of the few who can pull it off. Notice that the stem and leaf plot is actually a histogram, although it retains the individual values and allows for easy visual comparisons between groups.

Not all distributions are symmetric; in fact, many are not. When we look at a frequency distribution, we may see a trailing off to one side or the other, as in Figure 8-5. This trait is called *skew*. A positively skewed frequency distribution trails to the right, a negative one to the left.

A type of graph known as the *boxplot* (or *box and whisker* plot) is useful for summarizing the shape of a skewed distribution. This takes advantage of the percentile scale. The data points are organized by rank and then divided into quarters, so that each quartile contains one-fourth of the total data points. In a skewed distribution, there will be an equal number of points on either side of the 50th percentile value but the spread will be different on either side. The 25th percentile will not be the same distance from the middle as is the 75th percentile.

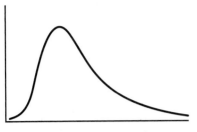

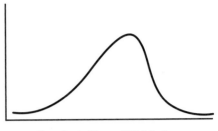

Positively Skewed Distribution   Negatively Skewed Distribution

FIGURE 8-5 Examples of data with skewed distributions.

- *The percentile scale uses markers that divide the total number of observations into equal parts.*

In a boxplot, the box encloses half of the data points, from the 25th to the 75th percentile. The horizontal line represents the median value, or 50th percentile. The lines that project from the box, the "whiskers," represents the rest of the values—those not close to the center. A potential limitation of this type of plot is the inability to detect more than one cluster. A stemplot would be more informative for these situations. Extreme values (*outliers*) are identified as points beyond the whiskers. Boxplots are ideal for a quick visual summary of the overall distribution. An advantage is their ability to present comparisons when they are placed side-by-side, as in Figure 8-6.

Outliers are data points that deviate unexpectedly from the others. These so-called red flags should raise suspicion if they are extreme and alone. They may reflect a problem with data collection or entry. Outliers should not be automatically discarded but they should be scrutinized for error since they have the potential to influence the validity of the results of the analysis.

These graphs illustrate some of the visual ways to portray distributions. They show us the pattern of variability and clustering, and are also a good way to scan for outliers. Distributions help statisticians decide what type of statistical test should be used in the final analysis. In addition to the type of variable and scale of measurement, the type of distribution of the variable is thus taken into consideration.

NUMERIC DESCRIPTORS OF A DISTRIBUTION

When we use biostatistics to make comparisons between groups, we use formulas to do the calculations. The actual values of the variable are needed in the process, so the data are compressed into *descriptors* that describe the shape of the distribution. We need to have a way to mathematically describe a variable's distribution so the calculations can be done. We know that, in nature, most variables have two attributes that account for the overall shape of a distribution:

1. They tend to cluster. This appears as a hill in a histogram or a big slice in a pie chart.
2. They vary. They have a range of values. The spread of values can be wide or narrow.

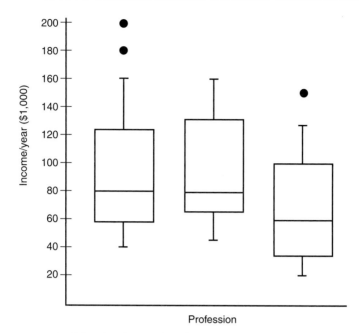

FIGURE 8-6 Box and whisker plot of reported yearly income for three professions. These graphs plot the yearly income × $1,000 for college graduates with three different degrees. The median values are the lines through the boxes. The overall range is the same, but shifted to less income for the third type of training. The first and third graphs show outliers who earn much more than the others.

There can be a few aberrant outlying values, which stand out visually toward the ends of a pictorial display. These two attributes can each be described by using numbers, which can then be used in the formulas.

MEASURES OF CENTRAL TENDENCY

There are three mathematical ways to describe the location of a cluster.

The *mode* describes the highest point of a hill in a frequency distribution. A distribution with a single hill is referred to as a unimodal distribution. There may be more than one hill; a trimodal distribution, for example, has three hills. In a unimodal distribution, the mode is the value that occurs most frequently. This measure is useful in describing nominal data.

- *MOde = MOst often*

Figure 8-7 shows the age distribution of reported tuberculosis cases in the United States by year of report: 1985, 1988, and 1991. The incidence of tuberculosis has a trimodal age distribution. Small children are affected, but not as much as young adults. There is another cluster in the elderly. We also see that in 1991 there was an increase in the incidence of tuberculosis in the most commonly affected age group, 30- to 40-year-olds.

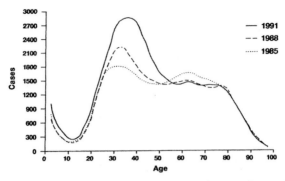

FIGURE 8-7 Age distribution of reported tuberculosis cases in the United States by year of report: 1985, 1988, and 1991. *(From Kent, J. H. 1993. The epidemiology of multidrug-resistant tuberculosis in the United States. Medical Clinics of North America, 77:6, 1393 with permission.)*

Many variables have distributions that tend to cluster around the middle value. The *median* value is the true midpoint. The number of values that are lower than this point equals the number of higher values. The median is also called the 50th percentile. This descriptor is used in rank type data (remember the ordinate scale? The differences between adjacent values is not consistent). It is also more representative of the middle value in a skewed distribution, such as we saw in Figure 8-5. When there is an odd number of observations, the median value is the one in the center after they are arranged in increasing value. If the number of observations is even, the median is the average of the two center observations. Figure 8-3 is a histogram that illustrates an uneven distribution where the median response is not the mode.

- *MeDian = MiDdle*

The *mean* of a distribution is the average value that is observed, symbolically shown as $\bar{X}$. The values are added up and the sum (represented by the symbol Σ) is divided by the number of observations. The formula is:

$$\text{Sample mean} = \frac{\text{sum of values of each observation in sample}}{\text{number of observations in sample}}$$

or, in mathematical terms,

$$\bar{X} = \frac{\Sigma X}{n}$$

where X represents each observation and n is the total number of observations.

- *MEAN = Multiple Entries, Average Number*

The median and mean will be close in value when the distribution is symmetrical. There is more play between these values when the distribution is skewed. The mean gets pulled toward the tail of the curve, as in Figure 8-8. The mean is a reliable measure

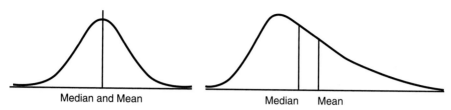

Median and Mean   Median   Mean

FIGURE 8-8 In a skewed distribution, the mean is pulled toward the tail of the curve.

of central tendency in a symmetric distribution. If there is skew, however, the median is a better measure of the center since it is less affected by extreme values or outliers.

MEASURES OF VARIABILITY

Just as there are mathematical descriptors for the cluster component of a distribution, the range or spread can also be described. It is apparent that, for any distribution, there will be many values that do not equal the mode, median, or mean. We can start by describing the range of values, from lowest to the highest. Some excessive values (the outliers) may pull the edge of the range to the extreme, which would not accurately reflect the overall closeness of most of the variables to the cluster.

A more reliable descriptor would be the average distance of all the values from the cluster. This is called the *standard deviation*. The difference between each value and the mean is calculated and the values are then averaged.

Since the mean is near the middle of the values, when the difference between each value and the mean is calculated, about half the numbers will be negative. When they are added together, the values will cancel each other and the total sum will be 0! This conundrum is avoided by squaring all the differences before adding them together, which ensures they will all be positive values. After they are added together, the sum is divided by the total number of observations, minus 1. The reason for this can be shown through complex mathematical arguments, but can be explained intuitively as our way of compensating for less variability in the sample than would be seen in the total population. This is referred to as the *variance*, s^2, of a distribution. The final step takes the square root of the variance to get the standard deviation, s.

For those interested, the formulas are shown here:

$$\text{Sample standard deviation} = \sqrt{\frac{\text{sum of (value of observation in the sample} - \text{sample mean})^2}{\text{number of observations in sample} - 1}}$$

or, in mathematical terms,

$$s = \sqrt{\frac{\sum (x_i - \bar{x})^2}{n-1}}$$

The standard deviation is useful when the distribution is symmetric but is less reliable in a skewed distribution. When there is skew, the variability is not consistent on either side of the median and there is really no "standard" deviation. In this case, it is more appropriate to use quartiles as descriptors of variability, as in the boxplot example. Outliers can also affect the standard deviation. A few aberrant values can have a great impact on the value of *s*.

The pattern of distribution of a variable is one of the determining factors when deciding what type of statistical test is appropriate for the data analysis. It is customary to graphically plot the data before performing the analysis to check for symmetry and scan for outliers.

When we want to study the effect of an intervention, for example, we take a sample group that is representative of the population we would like to study. Statisticians make a distinction between the mean and standard deviation of a variable from the sample (which is easy to measure) and those of the population (which can often only be estimated). Recall that the sample measurements are called *statistics*, which estimate these population *parameters*. The sample statistics are designated by Roman letters. The sample mean is denoted by $\overline{X}$ and the sample standard deviation is *s*. They are estimates of the population parameters, which use Greek letters. The population mean is designated by μ, whereas the population standard deviation uses the symbol sigma (σ).

	Population parameter	is estimated by	*Sample statistic*
Mean	μ (pronounced "mew")		$\overline{X}$
Standard Deviation	σ (sigma)		*s*

PARAMETRIC AND NONPARAMETRIC TESTS

When certain types of data are plotted on a frequency distribution, they will not display symmetry. Also, certain variables (e.g., categorical ones) are not measured in interval scales. These types of data are often analyzed with tests that do not make assumptions about the symmetry of the distribution of the variable. These are called *nonparametric tests*, or *distribution-free techniques*. The graph in Appendix A illustrates how the distribution of these variables can affect the type of statistical test that is ultimately used. In general, the nonparametric methods are easier to use but are considered more crude than parametric tests and are less sensitive at picking up significant effects. They are frequently used, however, because many types of data do not satisfy the symmetrical distribution required for parametric testing.

TYPES OF BIOSTATISTICS

We were introduced to the concepts of descriptive and inferential statistics in Chapter 1. Since we have now expanded our statistical vocabulary, we can look at the distinctions between these using a more formal definition. The above distributions represent the spread of all the values of a single variable. There are no comparisons being made between different groups within the population, or among variables. The graphs are informative but we cannot draw any conclusions about differences or similarities regarding other groups.

- *Descriptive statistics describe the variables in a data set.*

Descriptive statistics can be used to eyeball the distribution of a variable. This determines the type of statistical test used in making comparisons, but descriptive statistics cannot tell us whether one pathway is better than another or if there is a relationship between variables. These types of questions are answered using inferential statistics.

- *Inferential statistics compares the values of variables in a data set so conclusions can be drawn.*

A recent newspaper article reviewed the effect of graduated licensing programs on new driver safety.[1] These programs first grant a provisional driver's license, which (among other restrictions) requires parental supervision. The journalist noted that these programs seemed to be working—three states had reported reduced accident rates involving new drivers since the program was introduced. However, a total of 38 states have introduced these types of programs. Did the three states have a better outcome because of the programs, or could this have happened due to chance alone? To find the answer, we need to be able to estimate the probability that we would have seen the same results if these programs did *not* make a difference. In the next chapters we will find out how to do this by constructing a type of frequency distribution that plots the possible outcomes against their frequency of occurrence using the available data.

KEY POINTS

- A distribution is the pattern observed in a collection of values for a variable.
- A histogram is a bar graph that plots observed values on the abscissa and frequencies on the ordinate.
- A frequency distribution is a type of histogram that plots the values of a continuous variable on the abscissa and their relative frequency in the data set on the ordinate.
- Frequency distributions are used to represent the probability of a chance occurrence by plotting the value of a continuous outcome variable on the abscissa and the frequency which we would observe this outcome due to chance on the ordinate.
- The collection of values of a variable can be plotted in a visually satisfying distribution, but the eyeless computer needs mathematical descriptors of the collection of values to do the necessary calculations.
- Descriptors of distributions include markers of central tendency, such as mean, median, and mode.
- Markers of variability include standard deviation from the mean.
- Outliers are aberrant data points that should be scrutinized for error since they can impact the final analysis. They have a greater impact on the mean and standard deviation than on the median or mode.
- The percentile scale puts the values of a variable in order by their rank, then divides them into groups with equal numbers of data points.
- Percentile scales are especially useful for variables that use an ordinal scale or if there are valid outliers in the distribution that need to be left in.
- The sample mean $\bar{X}$ is an estimate of the population parameter μ.

- The sample standard deviation *s* is an estimate of the population parameter σ.
- Parametric tests are used for variables with distributions that fit certain criteria, such as symmetry and interval scales of measurement; otherwise, nonparametric tests can be used, although they are less sensitive overall at picking up significant effects.

REFERENCE

1. Durbin, D. 2003. Graduated licensing is working. Flint, MI: *The Flint Journal*, February 18.

REVIEW QUESTIONS

1. The _____ of a variable is a visual display of all the _____ of that variable.

2. Many types of variables have values that tend to cluster. The measures of central tendency include the _____, _____, and _____.

3. A measure of variability is the _____ _____.

4. An outlier has more effect on the _____ than on the median.

5. The sample mean and standard deviation are _____ of the population parameters.

True or False:

6. In any distribution, there will always be an individual value equal to the mode.

7. In any distribution, there will always be an individual value equal to the mean.

8. In any distribution, there will always be an individual value equal to the median.

ANSWERS TO REVIEW QUESTIONS

1. distribution, values

2. mean, median, mode

3. standard deviation

4. mean

5. estimates

True or False:

6. True

7. False

8. True if total number of observations is odd; may be false if total number of observations is even.

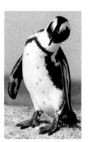

CHAPTER 9

The Normal Distribution

The process begins with the bell curve, the main purpose of which is to indicate not accuracy but error.

—*Peter L. Bernstein*[1]

There is a distinct type of frequency distribution that occurs naturally in many types of biologic data, especially variables that follow a continuous or interval scale. It is also one of the most commonly used distributions in statistics because it portrays the relative frequency with which a particular outcome could occur in many types of situations. For this reason, it is used as a prototype to demonstrate how the process of inferential statistics works.

The normal distribution was originally presented by the French mathematician Abraham de Moivre (1667–1754). He realized that to use samples to represent much larger populations, as Jacob Bernoulli had suggested, a pattern must emerge from the data. He demonstrated that the values of a variable in a sample would be distributed around the average value. When he plotted the values in a frequency distribution, the result was a unimodal and symmetric curve. The data points were distributed equally on either side of the mean. The ends tailed off toward the abscissa because the values farthest from the mean value were less likely to occur. This is called a *normal* distribution, since de Moivre attributed this pattern to the orderliness of the natural world. The famous mathematician Carl Friedrich Gauss expounded on this distribution, so it also became known as the Gaussian distribution. Figure 9-1 shows that it has a graceful bell shape, and thus is sometimes referred to as the *bell curve*.

ATTRIBUTES OF THE NORMAL DISTRIBUTION

There is a mathematical equation for the normal distribution that describes the relationship between the points on the abscissa and the ordinate. A collection of values with a normal distribution will have a mean μ and standard deviation σ. These descriptors determine the peak of the curve and its spread. There are many different bell curves for different values of μ and σ. For a particular curve, however, the height of the curve y at any given point depends on the value of x. Box 9–1 shows the formula for normal distributions, but it is not necessary to memorize it.

FIGURE 9-1 The normal distribution has a characteristic bell shape.

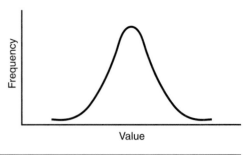

BOX 9-1

The formula for a normal distubution is :

$$y = \frac{1}{\sigma\sqrt{2\pi}} \exp\left[-\frac{1}{2}\left(\frac{X-\mu}{\sigma}\right)^2 \right]$$

All of the values on the right side of the equation are known except for x, because they are determined from the data (π is a constant). So, for any value of x along the abscissa we can solve for y, which is the frequency at which it occurs.

In a normal distribution, the mode is the peak of the hill. It is the value that occurs most frequently. It is also the mean, or the average of all the values in the distribution that is represented by μ. And because the data points are evenly distributed on either side, the same point represents the median, which is the 50th percentile. When μ changes but σ remains the same, the curve will shift along the abscissa but the shape remains the same, as in Figure 9-2.

Figure 9-3 shows what happens to the overall shape of the curve for different values of σ. When the standard deviation is smaller, the average distance from the mean is less, so more data points will have a value closer to the mean. This results in a narrower curve with a higher peak. The mean stays the same, but the curve is drawn upward.

We see that the normal distribution is actually a collection of bell-shaped curves, depending on μ and σ. We will ultimately use the curve as a frequency distribution

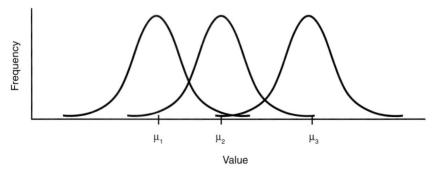

FIGURE 9-2 The effect of different values of μ with the same value of σ.

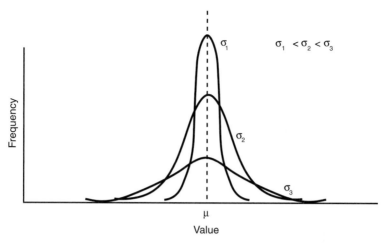

FIGURE 9-3 In a normal distribution the mode = mean = median = 50th percentile = μ. If the standard deviation is σ small, the curve is narrow and tall. As σ gets larger the curve gets shallow and wide.

to plot outcomes on the abscissa, so we can see the probability of their occurrence on the ordinate. It is to our advantage to somehow standardize all of these curves so we only need to refer to one. We can do this by performing some simple mathematical alterations to each data point. It is possible because the family of normal distributions are related by the way the data points are arranged under portions of the curve.

One of the distinctions of the normal distribution is related to its symmetry. One half of the data points lie to the left of μ and the remaining half lie to the right, no matter how spread out they are. When we plot all the data points, we also find that 68% of all of the observations fall within one standard deviation (σ) from the mean. When we go out two standard deviations on either side of the mean (actually 1.96 standard deviations, but often approximated to 2), about 95% of all observations will be encompassed in this area. The same distance (or deviation) from the mean will roughly contain the same number of data points on either side. In fact, one method to check for normality of data is to compute the percentile points in a collection of values for a variable and see if roughly 68% and 95% of the values fall within one and two standard deviations, respectively.

Figure 9-4 is an illustration of this principle. The population mean μ is also the median, and marks the 50th percentile. One half of the data points live on either side of μ. When going out one standard deviation (σ) on either side, the markers are at the 16th and 84th percentiles. This means 68% of the data points lie between these two markers (84 − 16 = 68). Likewise, the markers for 95% of the data points are 97.5 and 2.5. When the points in the two tails of the graph outside these markers are excluded, 95% of the original data points will be housed here.

This is an important distinction, especially when using these graphs to calculate probability. Even though it is correct to say that 95% of the data points live *below* the 95th percentile, probability calculations often use the data points *between* two markers that are the same distance in standard deviations from the mean. Figure 9-5 shows that the area under any normal distribution that encompasses 95% of the data points

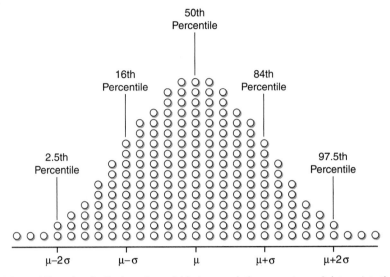

FIGURE 9-4 When the distribution of a variable is normal, the percentage of data points that fall within one or two standard deviations is always the same, no matter what the value of σ or μ. *(From Glantz, S. A. 1992. Primer of biostatistics, 3rd ed. New York: McGraw-Hill, p. 20, with permission.)*

is plus and minus 1.96 standard deviations. This corresponds to the 2.5th and 97.5th percentile markers. As we shall see, this distinction is the basic principle behind one-tailed and two-tailed tests.

THE STANDARDIZED NORMAL DISTRIBUTION

All normal distributions have the same overall shape, although the height of the peak may vary and the spread between the percentile markers may be different from one

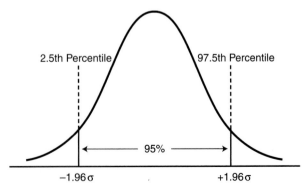

FIGURE 9-5 The area between the 2.5th and 97.5th percentile markers contain 95% of the data points in any normal distribution. These points can be found at ± 1.96 σ.

normal distribution to the other. However, the markers of the 68th and 95th percentiles (which encompass approximately 68% and 95% of the total data points, respectively) will still be located at about the first and second standard deviation values. This attribute allows for a *standardization* of any normal distribution. We can define the distance along the abscissa in terms of standard deviations from the mean instead of the true value of the data point. This condenses all normal distributions into one through a mathematical manipulation of the data.

Each data point is converted into a standardized value, and its new value is referred to as a *Z* score:

$$Z = \frac{X - \mu}{\sigma}$$

The new value, or *Z* score, corresponds to the number of standard deviations from the mean. When these are plotted, the standardized normal distribution results, as in Figure 9-6. Any normal distribution can be standardized in this way.

- *In any normal distribution, the scale along the x-axis can be transformed into standard deviations from the mean, without changing the relative shape of the curve. This is called standardization.*

The standardized normal distribution has a mean of 0 and a standard deviation of 1. This standardized normal distribution refers to the data points in terms of distance

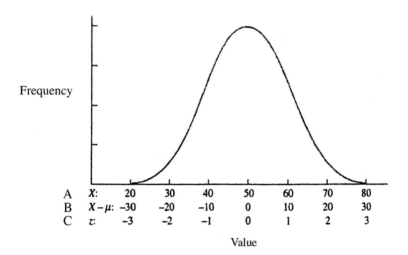

		20	30	40	50	60	70	80
A	*X*:	20	30	40	50	60	70	80
B	$X - \mu$:	−30	−20	−10	0	10	20	30
C	*z*:	−3	−2	−1	0	1	2	3

Value

Original data: $\mu = 50$ $\sigma = 10$
Standardized data: $\mu = 0$ $\sigma = 1$

FIGURE 9-6 In the standardized normal distribution, $\mu = 0$. Each value of *x* is standardized to the mean (μ) by subtracting μ from *x*, as in line B. In the standardized normal distribution, $\sigma = 1$. Each value is then standardized to σ when it is divided by the value of σ, as in line C. Now each data point is fully standardized and has a new value called the *Z* score. *(Adapted from Howell, D. C. 1999. Fundamental statistics for the behavioral sciences, 4th ed. Pacific Grove, CA: Brooks/Cole Publishing Co., p. 93, with permission.)*

from the mean, or standard deviations. Once we know the mean and standard deviation of a normal distribution, we can calculate the Z score for any value of x.

- A Z score is the number of standard deviations above or below the mean in a standardized normal distribution.

If $Z = 1$, that is one standard deviation from the mean in the positive direction on the right. If $Z = -2.5$, that is 2.5 standard deviations from the mean on the left. The mean, by definition, has no deviation, so its Z score is 0. The way the data points are distributed is the same for any normal distribution, and now the percentile markers can be expressed in terms of Z.

HOW TO USE A Z SCORE

We are now ready to do a simple problem using descriptive data that illustrates an application of the normal distribution. Over many years of data collection, we know that the human intelligence quotient (IQ) is measured on a continuous scale with a mean of 100 and standard deviation of 15, and that it has a normal distribution. If you know an individual's IQ, you can convert it to a Z score and find the corresponding percentile rank for that individual by consulting a Z table. For an IQ of 105, the conversion would be:

$$Z = \frac{x - \mu}{\sigma} = \frac{105 - 100}{15} = \frac{5}{15} = 0.33$$

This individual test score is 0.33 standard deviations above the mean. (A negative Z score would be below the mean.) To convert to percentile, we need to consult a table that gives us the relative areas for portions of the standardized normal distribution. Appendix C has an abbreviated Z table. It shows only the positive Z scores—those to the right of the mean. The first column represents the values for Z to the first decimal, in this case 0.3. Follow this row until you find the area for $Z = 0.33$. The area is 0.1293. To find the total area, we need to add 0.5 for the area to the left of the mean. This results in a total of 0.6293, rounded to 0.63. The percentile ranking of a person who scores 105 on the IQ test is 63%. S/he has scored better than 62.9% of all those who take the test.

A little manipulation is necessary to find the percentile ranking for the lower part of the curve, or the values less than 100. Because the curve is symmetric, only half the scores really need to be published; the rest can be derived using so-called mirror image techniques. For details on how this is done, consult one of the listed references.

THE NORMAL DISTRIBUTION AS A PREDICTOR OF EVENTS

Standardization is used to convert normal distributions containing data points into a more usable distribution to calculate probability. Remember that the normal distribution is a frequency distribution, so that the height of the curve at any point represents the relative frequency of that value. Because each data point represents an observation, if we randomly picked one point from the data set we could actually estimate the chances that the point would have a given value. We know, for instance, that any randomly picked value has a 95% chance of falling within 1.96 standard deviations from the mean.

If you are familiar with calculus you will recognize that the area under a curve can be calculated mathematically. The normal distribution gives us a shortcut. Once we standardize, we can convert any data point into a Z score. This property allows us to consult a single table to find these areas once we are working in the standardized normal distribution. We could use calculus to find the areas using the formula of the normal distribution, but standardizing to Z and using a published table is easier by far.

The Z table is useful for calculating percentiles for individuals when the mean and standard deviation of the population are known. However, many statistical procedures test for difference between groups rather than focusing on an individual. For example, we are more interested in a medical intervention that provides an overall advantage to the *average* individual of the group rather than to a singular individual. This type of approach uses parameters that are based on sample means rather than an individual value. We will see how the mean of a variable from a sample uses the normal distribution in this process. We will also see that normal distributions can be applied to skewed distributions when we take many samples and plot their means.

The normal distribution, it turns out, has many direct applications in statistics. We have seen how the standardized normal distribution allows us to calculate probability. Many statistical tests use this distribution in an analogous fashion to test for significance. Despite the fact that it resembles a spineless jellyfish, the normal distribution has distinguished itself as the backbone of inferential statistics. Not only does it represent the pattern of many naturally occurring variables, it is also the mathematical model of numerous probability calculations that are used in predicting outcomes.

The normal distribution will be used as the prototype model in this book to illustrate the concepts behind inferential statistics. This elegant curve depicts the probability of events, which leads us to inference.

KEY POINTS

- The normal distribution is a frequency distribution that occurs commonly in nature.
- It is unimodal and symmetric. Its mean = median = mode = 50th percentile. Its ends taper off into infinity on either side of the mean.
- In all normal distributions, 68% of the values fall within 1 standard deviation, and 95% of the values fall within 2 (actually 1.96) standard deviations.
- The area under the normal curve is directly related to probability.
- If a value were picked at random, there would be a 95% chance that it would fall between the 2.5th and 97.5th percentiles (± 1.96 standardized deviations from the mean).
- If we obtained a random value and wondered whether it was from a certain distribution, and when it was plotted on the abscissa it was below the 2.5th percentile, we would conclude it is very unlikely that the value came from that distribution (although that could happen less than 2.5% of the time).
- The standardized normal distribution converts all values into Z scores. These are standard deviation units. The mean value will have a Z score of 0 since it

does not deviate at all from the mean. The standard deviation of the original distribution takes on a value of 1.

■ The standard normal distribution has an area equal to 1 under its curve. Any portion of the curve thus has a value between 0 and 1.

■ Instead of doing calculus to find the area of a normal distribution, we standardize it so that we use a single table (based on the Z score) to find the area of a portion of the curve which translates into probability.

REFERENCE

1 Bernstein, P. L. 1988. *Against the gods: The remarkable story of risk.* New York: John Wiley & Sons, Inc., p. 141.

REVIEW QUESTIONS

1. Many types of variables in nature have values that, when plotted on a _____ _____, take on the shape of a normal distribution.

2. In a normal distribution, _____% of the data points lie between the 2.5th and 97.5th percentile markers. In a normal distribution, _____% of the data points lie between −1.96 and +1.96 standard deviations.

3. When we standardize a normal distribution, we know that now _____% of the data points lie between $Z = +1.96$ and −1.96.

4. The area under a portion of any normal distribution can be found using _____ methods.

5. It is a much simpler approach to convert a value from a normal distribution to a Z score and consult a table that lists the area on either side of that score for the _____ normal distribution.

6. For an IQ score of $Z = 0$, the percentile ranking is _____.

7. When applied to outcomes, the area under a normal distribution correlates with the _____ of an event occurring.

8. The standardized normal distribution has an area equal to _____ under its curve.

9. If $Z = 0$, this places the data point right on the _____ of the standardized normal distribution.

10. If you were to randomly choose a standardized value from the normal distribution, the value most likely to occur would be $Z =$ _____.

11. For a randomly chosen single value from a standardized normal distribution, one with a Z score of −3 would be very _____ to occur.

ANSWERS TO REVIEW QUESTIONS

1. frequency distribution

2. 95, 95

3. 95

4. calculus

5. standardized

6. 50th

7. probability

8. 1

9. mean, mode, and median

10. 0

11. unlikely

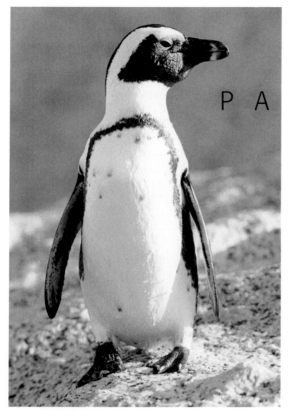

Understanding Inference

The ability to define what may happen in the future and to choose among alternatives lies at the heart of contemporary society

—*Peter L. Bernstein*[1]

INTRODUCTION TO PART II

Inferential statistics can tell us, with a certain degree of confidence, if there is a true difference between two pathways, or if the difference is likely due to chance outcomes. It's also used to determine the likelihood of a true relationship between two or more variables. We use a sample to represent the population, and only one sample at that. We know that each sample will give a different result, but we are willing to accept a degree of uncertainty so we don't have to observe each member of the population.

To illustrate the degree of faith required to accept a result as valid, consider the scenario so eloquently stated by Stanton Glantz in Figure II-1.

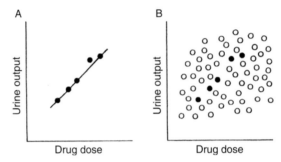

FIGURE II-1 (A) Results of an experiment in which researchers administered five different doses of a drug to five different people and measured their daily urine production. Output increased as the dose of drug increased in these five people, suggesting that the drug is an effective diuretic in all people similar to those tested. (B) If the researchers had been able to administer the drug to all people and measure their daily urine output, it would have been clear that there is no relationship between the dose of drug and urine output. The five specific individuals who happened to be selected for the study in panel A are shown as shaded points. It is possible, but not likely, to obtain such an unrepresentative sample that leads one to believe that there is a relationship between the two variables when there is none. A set of statistical procedures called tests of hypotheses permits one to estimate the chance of getting such an unrepresentative sample. *(From Glantz, S. A. 1992.* Primer of Biostatistics, *3rd ed. New York, NY: McGraw-Hill, pp. 5-6.)*

The moral behind this story is that there really is no true effect between the drug dose and the urine output, which would have been apparent if we could have studied the entire population. It was purely bad luck that we chose a sample that led us to believe in a true diuretic effect of the drug. The point to be emphasized, however, is that it would be extremely unlikely that we would choose such a random sample. It could happen by chance, but it's overwhelmingly more likely our sample would more accurately represent the lack of drug effect that would be observed in the population.

Samples do not act irrationally. They are governed by predictable patterns of behavior. They may go awry once in a blue moon but they will most often follow the rules if they have been chosen according to the laws of random selection. Become comfortable with this fact. Then you will be able to depend on the sample data to provide you with a reliable conclusion.

REFERENCE

1. Bernstein P. L. 1998. *Against the gods*, New York: John Wiley & Sons, Inc., p. 7.

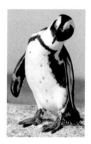

CHAPTER 10

Hypothesis Testing

Alert human beings, hit by something unpleasant, seek to find its cause so that they can avoid it in the future.

—*Robert Hooke*[1]

We know that the values of many variables that occur in nature have a Gaussian or bell-shaped frequency distribution. The height of the curve is lowest at the tail ends, so those values do not occur very frequently. If we were to pick a value at random from this distribution, it would be very unlikely that the value would be from one of the ends of the distribution; it is much more likely to be from somewhere toward the middle.

In the same way, if an event takes place that has multiple possible outcomes, and the outcome variable has a normal frequency distribution, certain outcomes are more likely to occur than others. The probability that a specific outcome will occur by chance depends on where in the normal frequency distribution it is located. The more likely outcomes are toward the middle, with higher values on the ordinate. Those less likely to occur will be at the tail ends of the distribution. A value picked at random will be very likely to be from the center portion of the graph.

Let us see how we can apply the logic of probability using the normal distribution to decide how likely it is that a medical intervention makes a real difference. Inferential statistics gives us the means to answer questions such as: Is one pathway better than another, on average? More specifically, we can answer these types of questions:

1. Is there a significant difference in the proportion of a variable in one of the groups?
2. Is the treatment or intervention more beneficial than another pathway, such as the current standard of care?
3. Are two variables linked?
4. Does one variable have an effect on another variable (such as the outcome)? What is the strength of effect?

These are very representative of the types of questions posed in research studies. The questions look at different problems but the overall approach to getting an answer is the same. The type of statistical test that is used is different, as is shown by the flow diagrams in Appendices A and B. The specific test depends on the type of variable and the question being asked. However, the logic behind the tests uses the same standard approach. We will look at each of these situations in more detail by focusing on the type of statistical test. Before we delve into the individual situations, however, we first need to understand the format that is used when performing statistical tests.

When a researcher sets up a clinical trial, s/he follows a basic protocol. These steps are common to every study even though the particular type of study may vary. These include the procedural steps as well as the logistic steps of the statistical process that focuses on hypothesis testing, which are in italics in the following list. We have discussed many of these concepts already, and are now ready to look at the statistical methodology.

- State the research hypothesis. This is a pertinent question that can be answered.
- Define the population and variables to be studied.
- Identify outcome variable, if applicable, and statistical test to be used.
- *State the null hypothesis.*
- *Declare significance level.*
- Estimate the number of subjects needed to get a reliable answer.
- Obtain appropriate committee approval and financing.
- Obtain a sample.
- Collect data.
- *Obtain the test statistic using the statistical method based on type of variables and type of question being asked.*
- *Apply the test statistic to a sampling distribution.*
- *Obtain p value.*
- *Make a decision to accept or reject the null hypothesis.*
- Derive a conclusion that answers the research hypothesis.

There is virtually an infinite number of topics that could potentially be studied. Not all research questions are answerable, however. Many questions are just too broad to be considered as a research hypothesis. Most major investigators will choose a topic in their field of expertise so they are able to pose questions that are particularly appropriate, given the prior research leading up to what is currently known about a subject. They are able to identify the next logical step in the process that leads to a usable understanding of the knowledge. They are aware of time and cost limitations when determining the feasibility of a research proposal. Ethical issues need to be considered, too. Many studies cannot be justified because they could be construed to take advantage of a certain group of people, especially those in lower socioeconomic classes or those who cannot give consent, such as a fetus.

The first step in research, then, is choosing an answerable question (keeping in mind the above constraints). Once that is done, the population to be studied is identified, as are the variables pertinent to the research hypothesis. The next step is to declare the null hypothesis, to see whether the data collected will support it. We cannot reach a conclusion unless we have gone this route.

THE NULL HYPOTHESIS AND ALTERNATIVE HYPOTHESIS

All statistical tests start out with the premise that the data are a result of chance variation. This hypothesis is called the *null hypothesis*, or H_0. This is different from the *research hypothesis*, which is the question that the experiment was designed to answer.

The null hypothesis is the first step in the actual process that is used in the statistical analysis.

In the first two types of research questions that were posed above, we are actually asking whether there is a difference between two or more groups with respect to the variable of interest, such as outcome. Another way of stating this is "Is it likely that the groups are different with respect to the intervention, or is the difference more likely due to chance?" The null hypothesis in this case would state that the treatment had no effect.

There will always be a difference when comparing the outcome variables of groups within a sample, because that is the nature of variables. They vary. So what we are really asking is "Does the difference of the outcome variable in the sample fall outside of the expected range when no difference really exists in the population?"

Besides testing for differences between groups exposed to alternate pathways, we can also use biostatistics to test for relationships between variables. The questions that would be posed in these circumstances would be similar to the above questions 3 and 4. The way to answer this type of question is to ask "How probable is it that the relationship we observed was due solely to chance variation in the value of the variables?" In this case, the null hypothesis (H_0) would state that there is no relationship between the variables in the population, and the statistical test used would test the likelihood that any apparent relationship was due to chance occurrence in the sample.

- *The null hypothesis, symbolized as H_0, states that there is no difference or no relationship among groups.*

In theory, *any* result we get is possible due to chance variation. Assuming that the result we observe is truly due to chance, we would like to know how probable it is that this could happen. If it is highly improbable to get the result we did if there is no true difference (or relationship) in groups, we will reject the null hypothesis as being too outlandish. Statistical methods used to test the null hypothesis are termed *tests of significance*, which we will talk about more in the next chapter.

Why do we use null hypothesis? It may seem like backward logic to assume that the outcomes are not dependent upon an intervention, and then to try to prove yourself wrong. Why not assume that there is a true difference and try to prove yourself right? The philosophical reasoning behind this approach was proposed by Fisher in the early 1900s, who developed the concept of hypothesis testing. Simply put, his argument states that it is easier to reject a statement as false by finding data that do not support it. However, to accept that something is always true, one must account for every instance in which the statement could be true. We would have to test multiple hypotheses—looking at every possible numerical relationship that could exist—which is an impossible task. It is therefore much more productive to form a statistical hypothesis of no difference or no relationship and then see if the data support or go against this hypothesis. Without delving into the specifics of the precise argument in favor of the null hypothesis, it is important to know that it is a starting point for virtually any statistical test. The logic of applied biostatistics is based on the null hypothesis, and it is widely accepted as the foundation of statistical testing.

It is customary to state an alternative hypothesis, which would be accepted if the null hypothesis were shown to be highly unlikely. In this case, we would reject the null hypothesis of no difference (or relationship) and adopt the alternative hypothesis that a treatment difference (or relationship among variables) does indeed exist. The typical symbol for the alternative hypothesis is H_a. Occasionally the symbol H_1

will be used. The specific alternative hypothesis depends on the question being asked. We will see examples of this in the following chapters.

- *The alternative hypothesis, symbolized as H_a or H_1, is adopted when the null hypothesis is rejected. It is the hypothesis of an existing difference or relationship, and often echoes the research hypothesis.*

If the data do not support a decision to reject the null hypothesis, then that is all we can say. We cannot state that the null hypothesis is true, only that is has not been rejected. Similar to a jury trial that attempts to prove guilt beyond a reasonable doubt, the data are used to establish a real treatment difference beyond reasonable doubt. Absence of guilt does not prove innocence, and absence of data to reject the null hypothesis does not prove it is true.

DATA ANALYSIS

The next step in the process of inference involves the specific type of statistical test to be used. This is an equation that is determined by the type of variable and its distribution. The data from the sample are entered into this equation and a single number emerges, which is referred to as the *test statistic*. This number has a direct connection with the p value. In the next chapter we will see exactly how test statistics are used to obtain p values. For now, it is helpful to think of the test statistic as a single number which is the result of the statistical analysis.

THE p VALUE

We have already been introduced to the concept of a p value as representing a probability, with a range of 0 (no probability of the event happening) to 100 (the event will always happen). Most probabilities fall somewhere between these extreme values.

The value of p represents the probability of an event occurring. In statistical testing, the p value is the probability that we would observe the result that we did if there is no true difference (or relationship, as was the case) between groups (that is to say, if the null hypothesis is correct.) If the p value is very low, that means the probability of seeing the result that we observed would be very unlikely if in fact no true difference existed between the groups. In this case we would reject the null hypothesis of no true difference, and adopt the alternative hypothesis of a true treatment difference.

- *The p value is the likelihood that the result observed is due to random occurrence, if H_0 is correct.*

The p value can be represented by the area under a curve. Therefore, it does not usually take on an exact value, but is more correctly used to denote a probability greater than or less than a given value. It is more correct to state "$p < 0.05$" rather than "$p = 0.05$."

THE SIGNIFICANCE LEVEL

A very logical question at this point is "If the p value can potentially take any value between 0 and 1, at what point do we draw the line and conclude that the results are too improbable to happen by chance alone?" A more specific way of stating this is "*What is the probability with which we are comfortable in rejecting the null hypothesis, even if it is correct?*" This level of comfort is referred to as the significance level. It is denoted by α.

- The significance level α is the value of p *at which we are willing to reject* H_0 *even if it is correct.*

Note that if we do decide to reject H_0 it is with the risk, albeit very small, of being wrong. Recall, however, that when using samples to study populations, the samples are *expected* to have some variation from the population (if we could measure every member of the latter). The samples are expected to be different from each other as well, since that is the nature of random sampling. We need to make a decision as to when the results observed are too improbable to support the null hypothesis. The most commonly accepted level of significance is $\alpha = 0.05$, or 5%. This means that the probability of observing the results we got, if there were truly no treatment effect (if the null hypothesis were true), is less than 5%. In other words, it is quite possible that we would be wrong in rejecting the null hypothesis, but it is not very likely since it would happen on the average only 5 times out of 100 (or 1 out of 20) over repeated experiments using different samples of the same size.

There is no scientific justification for the rather arbitrary significance level of 0.05. It feels very comfortable to many individuals (just as an ambient temperature of 72°F is by consensus a comfortable environment) and 0.05 has historically been adapted as the standard significance level for rejecting the null hypothesis. It is generally accepted that the risk of being wrong 1 out of 20 times is sufficiently stringent to prevent gross errors in medical management. When studies are repeated that support the observation of the first trial, then the evidence becomes overwhelmingly in favor of the original conclusion. There are also legal references to acceptable margins of error. *Castaneda v. Partida* was a 1976 case of alleged ethnic bias against Mexican Americans in jury selection. In its review of the case, the Supreme Court endorsed "two or three standard deviations" as a criterion for statistical significance.[2]

The general consensus is that when $p < 0.05$, there is a significant difference in the two pathways. The pathway with the better result is then felt to be superior by statistical techniques. A p value of <0.01 is even more supportive of a true difference due to an intervention. In general, the smaller the p value, the less likely the result was due to random occurrence and the less likelihood of error when we reject H_0.

The normal distribution can be considered a distribution of probabilities to illustrate the above concepts. When we used the standardized normal distribution, the Z score was applied to a table which gave us an area that was directly proportional to probability. We now can use an analogous situation to answer the types of questions we posed at the beginning of this chapter.

The p value is determined by a statistical test, which is specific to each type of variable and question. A p value that falls within the extreme tails of the graph is highly unlikely to occur due to chance if the null hypothesis is correct. In Figure 10-1, this represents the shaded areas. If a value fell within one of these areas, it could happen by chance less than 5% of the time.

This is a situation where the probability of occurrence follows a normal distribution. If our statistical test resulted in a value of $p < 0.15$, we see that this falls to the ends of the curve, but not extreme enough that we would feel comfortable in rejecting the null hypothesis. We would conclude that the two groups had no *significant* difference in outcome. We fail to reject the null hypothesis (that is like accepting the null

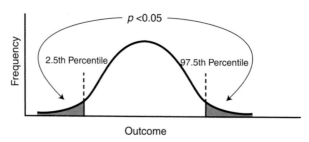

Outcome

FIGURE 10-1 The possible values of a test statistic are plotted on a frequency distribution. If the result falls to one of the shaded areas, the likelihood of obtaining this result due to chance alone is low, that is reflected in a low *p* value. Taken together the chance of seeing a result this extreme is <5%.

hypothesis of no treatment difference) and say that one treatment did not show an advantage over the other at the 0.05 significance level.

TYPES OF ERROR

If you are an individual who likes to be right on target, you may feel a little reluctant to take a chance on being wrong when using a *p* value to make a decision. Keep in mind, though, that inferential statistics is what it is. It uses the statistics to infer a conclusion. Inferential biostatistics is not 100% perfect, but the methodology is very reliable as long as we are willing to accept this small degree of possible error. There are potentially two ways we could err in our conclusion to reject or accept H_0. We could declare H_0 to be false when we get a small *p* value but, as you know, we could be wrong since a small *p* value could occur even when H_0 is true. In this case, we have inappropriately rejected H_0. When we claim a difference that does not exist, we are making a Type I error.

A Type II error, on the other hand, is accepting H_0 when it is in fact false, and H_a is true. We are missing a true treatment difference. As we will see, one scenario in which this can happen is when the sample size is too small to detect a significant difference, even when one exists. *Power calculations* are designed to minimize the chance that this will happen so that when no significant difference is detected and we do not reject H_0, it is very unlikely that we are making an error. Table 10-1 outlines the different types of errors in statistical decision making.

ONE- AND TWO-TAILED TESTS

Many studies look at differences in pathways or interventions. For instance, they may be studying the effect of a new drug on cancer patients, compared to the old drug that is the standard of care. The investigators may have an idea of what the results will be or which pathway may have a better outcome. If they are asking only whether one specific therapy is better than another, the research hypothesis might state "Does the new drug have a *better* outcome than the standard drug?"

TABLE 10-1 **Statistical Tests**

Decision based on data from sample	True State in Population	
	H_0 **True**	H_a **True**
Reject H_0	Type I error	No error
Accept H_0	No error	Type II error

The interpretation of statistical tests involves the acceptance of a small possibility of error. This "allowable error" is called alpha error when H_0 is true, and beta error when the H_a is true.

In most circumstances, however, it is quite feasible that the standard drug could turn out to be better. If this is not considered, then the investigators will not account for this possibility. Even if the standard drug is better, the test will show that there is no advantage either way. They (and ultimately we) would miss out on this potentially important knowledge. This is called a *one-tail test*, or a *directional test*. It is set up to reject H_0 in the instance that the result falls in only one of the tails of Figure 10-2.

- A one-tailed test, or directional test, accounts for a treatment difference in only one direction, even if the opposite is true.

Even though the researchers may suspect that the new drug is better, the possibility of a reverse outcome in favor of the defending champion standard drug should be accounted for. In fact, is that not why the study is being done in the first place? An unbiased approach that considers either possibility is called *equipoise*. The statistical test that reflects equipoise is called a *two-tailed test*, or *nondirectional* test. H_0 will be rejected if there is a result that falls at either tail, as in Figure 10-3.

- A two-tailed test, or nondirectional test, accounts for a treatment difference in either direction.

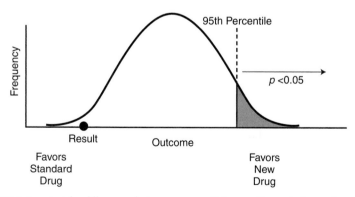

FIGURE 10-2 In a test for differences between groups, if the results are in favor of one pathway having a better outcome, the result will fall at one of the tails of the graph. In this case, the standard drug is better but this was missed because the test was constructed to pick up a difference only if the new drug was better. A 5% significance level was used.

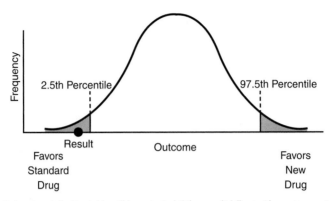

FIGURE 10-3 In a two-tailed test, H_0 will be rejected if the result falls at either extreme. The allowable error, or alpha error, must be divided between the two tails.

We reject H_0 if it seems too unlikely. If we adhere to the 5% significance level in a one-tailed test, we can apply the entire 5% error at one end of the graph. This means there are less stringent conditions to reject H_0 and declare a true treatment difference as compared to a two-tailed test. Figure 10-4 illustrates how a one-tailed test could result in a completely opposite conclusion from a two-tailed test with the same data.

Many statistical experts would agree that the rules of equipoise should be followed and, whenever possible, a two-tailed test should be done instead of a one-tailed test. However, it would not be unusual to encounter arguments that favor directional tests in certain circumstances, especially when prior research has supported directional results. There is no right or wrong approach, but the directional tests are more lenient in their ability to interpret a treatment difference because they apply all the "allowable uncertainty" to a circumstance that favors one particular outcome while ignoring the possibility of the other. Keep these opposing points of view in mind as you critique the literature.

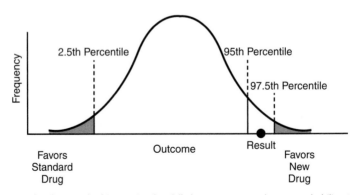

FIGURE 10-4 The data resulted in a point that falls between 5% and 2.5% probability. A two-tailed test would find in favor of H_0 and declare that there is no benefit for the new drug. A one-tailed test would be interpreted completely differently; H_0 would be rejected and the new drug would be declared significantly better.

STATISTICAL VERSUS CLINICAL SIGNIFICANCE

It is important to note that *statistical* significance may not always translate into *clinical* significance. It is possible through data mining to find statistical significance at many levels, especially in large databases with numerous variables. Very large sample sizes will tend to pick up statistically significant differences in variables, even if the difference is minute. If a pathway can be shown to be statistically advantageous, it is not necessarily a better way to go. Always consider what is being compared as well as the cost of treatment, the potential side effects, and the overall benefit to the population under study. If the clinical advantage is incrementally small, it may not justify the expense and effort to implement the change.

A MEMORY TRICK

Many of us who do not participate regularly in research cannot recall the accurate definition of a *p* value when we need to. That is understandable because the concept is somewhat complex. Here is an easy way to remember exactly what the *p* value represents:

- The *p* value is a probability. That is easy, because that is what *p* stands for.
- But, probability of what?
- Now that you have come this far in biostatistics, you are a "PRO." A PRO knows the definition of a *p* value. It is the Probability of a Random Occurrence.

That is most of it, but not all. Since I have "given" you this mnemonic, "give" me more detail:

- A *p* value is the Probability of a Random Occurrence, given that the null hypothesis is correct.

Now you are really a PRO!

KEY POINTS
- Inferential statistics can answer questions about relationships between variables or differences between groups.
- Research studies start out with a research hypothesis that should be a pertinent, answerable question.
- One of the common steps in the process of inference is hypothesis testing.
- Hypothesis testing starts with the null hypothesis, H_0, of no relationship or no difference.
- The statistical test that is done on the data depends on the type of question being asked and the types of variables being studied.
- The result of the statistical test is used to determine the *p* value.
- The *p* value is the probability of a random occurrence, given that the null hypothesis is correct.
- A small *p* value reflects a small chance of a random occurrence, and we reject the null hypothesis of no relationship or no difference as being too improbable and declare that there is a true difference between groups (as when an intervention works) or a true relationship between variables.

- The alternative hypothesis, H_a, is adopted if H_0 is rejected. It usually echoes the research hypothesis.
- The significance level is the value of p at which we are willing to reject H_0 even if it is correct. It is customary to use a 5% significance level, which corresponds to $p < 0.05$.
- We could be wrong in our decision to reject H_0. This is a Type I error.
- If we fail to reject H_0 when there *is* a true difference or true relationship, we are making a Type II error. Power calculations attempt to ensure that this type of error will not be a result of an inadequate sample size.
- A directional test is a one-tailed test that looks for a treatment advantage in one direction only.
- Equipoise is an attitude that makes no assumptions about the results before they have come in.

REFERENCES

1. Hooke, R. 1983. *How to tell the liars from the statisticians.* New York: Marcel Dekker, Inc., p. 137.
2. Moore D. S. and G. P. McCabe. 1999. *Introduction to the practice of statistics,* 3rd ed. New York: W. H. Freeman and Co., p. 619.

REVIEW QUESTIONS

1. The _____ _____ assumes there is no treatment benefit or relationship between variables.

2. If our test result is too incompatible with the null hypothesis, we _____ it and assume the _____ hypothesis is correct.

3. The statistical test ultimately results in a p value, which is the probability of a _____ _____, given that the null hypothesis is correct.

4. A _____-_____ test will consider a benefit of either pathway.

ANSWERS TO REVIEW QUESTIONS

1. null hypothesis

2. reject, alternative

3. random occurrence

4. two-tailed

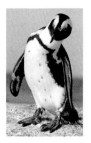

CHAPTER 11

The Probability Connection

Statistics are history, and we gather them so that we can learn from history. Usually what we can learn is how our chances of success depend on our actions.

—*Robert Hooke*[1]

We now know that *p* represents the probability of a chance occurrence. We also know that interpretation of the data, in every statistical test, centers around the *p* value and the probability of obtaining the result we saw if the null hypothesis of no effect is true. We know that probability can be represented graphically as a frequency distribution. We are now ready to see how *p* values are obtained. Even though different types of statistical tests are used, the overall logic is the same.

Various statistical methods are available that use different equations to obtain a *p* value. Since this is not an all-inclusive text on statistics, it is not sufficiently comprehensive if you are interested in statistical methodology. However, by the end of this chapter you will be familiar with some of the most commonly employed statistical methods.

SAMPLING DISTRIBUTIONS

One of the advantages of working with samples is that the investigator does not have to observe each member of the population to get the answer to the question being asked. A sample, when taken at random, represents the population. The sample can be studied and conclusions drawn about the population from which it was taken.

Let us focus on the group that makes up the sample. We are not as interested in an individual's response as we are in the group's response. The individual values, of course, are accounted for in the group, but the way to compare outcomes is by looking at an overall response. The data from the groups are used to estimate a parameter. As you recall, these are values that represent an average of a collection of values, such as average age or standard (which is really "average") deviation from the mean age.

To see how this is done, let us first look at a hypothetical situation. Consider what would happen if we were to study a population variable with a normal distribution. If we were to take multiple samples from this population, each sample theoretically would have a slightly different mean and standard deviation. When all sample means

($\overline{X}$s) are plotted (if this could be done), they would tend to cluster around the true population mean, µ. Many would even be right on the mark.

The problem, of course, is that we don't know *with certainty* how close we are by looking at just one sample. The mean of any given sample ($\overline{X}$) could be on either side of µ and at a different distance from µ.

Figure 11-1 illustrates what could happen when we take a sample from the population. This is a very clever idea that was used to illustrate the concept of sampling distributions in the *Primer of Biostatistics* by Stanton Glantz.[2] In this case, the population is Martians (as in those who are from Mars). Figure11-1A shows the frequency distribution for the heights in *every member* of the population, assuming this could be measured. But since we really cannot actually measure this, notice the various *samples* that were taken in graphs B, C, and D. The dots are the sample means; they are close but not exact. The bars on either side of the mean dots represent the samples' standard deviations.

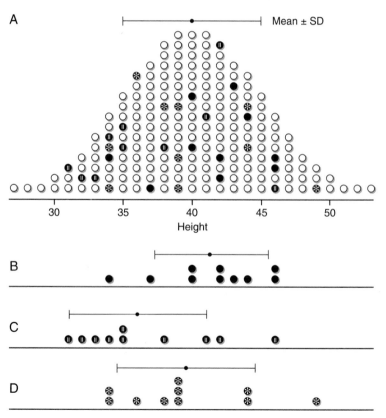

FIGURE 11-1 If one draws three different samples of 10 members each from a single population, one will obtain three different estimates of the population mean and standard deviation. *(From Glantz, S. A. 1992. Primer of biostatistics, 3rd ed. New York: McGraw-Hill, p. 23, with permission.)*

Now cover up graph A. The laws of random sampling tell us that each of these samples was equally likely to be picked. They are pretty good estimators for the population parameter of mean height. It is highly unlikely to pick a sample comprised of only members at one end of the curve. In this case, the estimate would be way off the mark.

Inferential statistics does not focus on "What is the true parameter?" Instead, we ask "How likely is it that we are within a certain distance from the true parameter?" What we really need to know is the degree of variability among the samples that could happen by chance, and the possibility of obtaining an aberrant or unusual sample. The method we use depends on *the sampling distribution of the test statistic.* Every statistical test relies on this. It is the basis of the entire theory of inference.

- *The sampling distribution of a statistic is the distribution of all values of that statistic for every sample of a particular size from the same population.*

The statistic in this case has a special meaning—it is the result of the data analysis that is used to estimate the population parameter. The sampling distribution is an abstract concept. The distribution of the sample statistic is the result of what would happen if every sample of a particular size were studied. Even though we study a single, random sample, it is only one of an incredibly large number of possible samples—each with its own statistic.

The rest of the chapter discusses how sampling distributions for different types of test statistics are generated. This is not an actual step in this process of inference testing. We do not create a distribution because we have only one sample to work with. The statisticians look at the sample size and the type and variability of the data to see which distribution to use.

In the above example, we talked about using a sample mean, designated as $\bar{X}$, to estimate the population parameter, μ. Many statistical tests will use sample means in the data analysis. There are other ways of analyzing data that result in different types of test statistics. We will explore a few of these as we look at different types of data but, for now, let us focus on just sample means as a way of estimating population means.

For any sample of a given size, we can calculate the mean, $\bar{X}$. If we were to plot the value of $\bar{X}$ on a frequency distribution, for all the values of $\bar{X}$ for samples of the same size, a pattern would emerge. The distribution of sample means has the same mean as the population but with a much smaller spread than the original sample. This makes sense because the means of each sample will not have the same degree of spread that the individual values do. The means plotted at the tails of the distribution will be less frequent, since a sample mean that deviates markedly from the population mean is very unlikely. Samples behave in a predictable fashion. They will have some variability but, if they come from the same population, the statistics will fall into a predictable collection of values. The *sampling distribution* is the illustration of this expected frequency and range.

Figure 11-2 is a graph of the means of 25 samples of Martian heights. When these means are plotted, a normal distribution emerges and forms a predictable pattern. Note that the mean of all of these samples, designated as $\bar{X}_{\bar{x}}$, is the same as the population mean, μ, but the spread of standard deviation of the means is much narrower than the original data. The deviation of the sample means (in this case, of 25 means) is known as the *standard error of the mean* to distinguish it from the standard

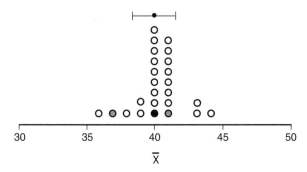

FIGURE 11-2 The frequency distribution of the sample means of the heights of Martians. *(From Glantz, S. A. 1992.* Primer of biostatistics, *3rd ed. New York: McGraw-Hill, p. 25, with permission.)*

deviation of a single sample. The standard error of the mean is denoted as $SE_{\bar{x}}$. As Glantz aptly states, "Unlike the standard deviation, which quantifies the variability in the population, the standard error of the mean quantifies uncertainty in the estimate of the mean."[3]

Theoretically, if we took the means for a given variable from every possible sample of the same size, we could plot these in a frequency distribution. Computer simulation actually can demonstrate this process. What emerges is a pattern that falls into the normal distribution, *even if the original distribution of the values was not normal.* Surprised? So was I at first. But it makes sense that sample *means* would tend to approach the true parameter, with equal chances of under- or overestimating the true mean.

Figure 11-3 is a computer-generated sampling distribution of means. The original population (graph A) had a mean of 50 and a standard deviation of 29. It was actually a rectangular distribution. All values between 0 and 100 were equally frequent.

In graphs B and C, each dot represents a sample mean. The means of the samples have a wider distribution for a smaller sample size of 5 (graph B), with an approximately normal distribution. When the sample size is increased to 30 (graph C), the distribution of the means is narrower.

It turns out that samples act in a predictable fashion. This predictability happens not only with sample means, but with other parameters as well. Recall that some parameters can be quite abstract, such as "risk of an accident." For all possible samples of the same size from a population, the risk calculated will form a predictable collection of values. The actual risk in the population is fixed and the sample provides you with an estimate of that risk.

Think of sampling distributions as predictable collections of numbers that form a pattern. The rest of the process then falls into place: if it is too unlikely that our sample statistic came from the predictable collection that we would expect if the treatment had no effect, we reject the null hypothesis and declare one treatment to be significantly better. The logic behind all the statistical tests is based on this method.

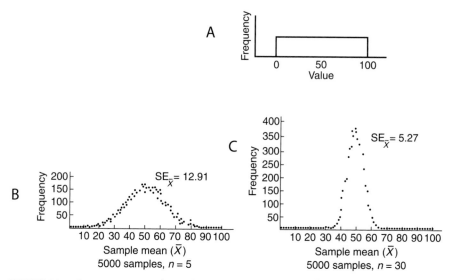

FIGURE 11-3 Computer-generated sampling distributions of means. *(From Howell, D. C. 1999. Fundamental statistics for the behavioral sciences, 4th ed. Pacific Grove, CA: Brooks/Cole Publishing Co., p. 226, with permission.)*

THE TEST STATISTIC

Data from a single sample can be analyzed for the mean or it can be looked at in other ways, which would depend on the type of variable(s) and the question being asked. These various analyses apply different types of equations that use the data to generate a single number. This number is known as the *test statistic*.

The test statistic, in itself, is meaningless. It is interpreted by its relative place on a frequency distribution of all possible test statistics that could result from all possible same-sized samples, if the null hypothesis were true. Its importance is determined by how far it lies from most of the test statistics we would expect to see if there were no treatment difference, or no relationship among variables.

- *The test statistic is a single number that assesses the compatibility of the data with the null hypothesis.*

The type of test to be used is dependent upon the type of variable(s) and question being asked. We apply the data to a specific equation. The actual analysis is usually done by computers, with programs that not only store the data but do the requested calculations. The result is a single number called the test statistic. For instance, a chi-square test for differences among groups results in a chi-square test statistic. A test for correlation results in a correlation coefficient, another type of test statistic. Some tests analyze differences in sample means, which results in a *t* statistic. We take this test statistic and apply it to a corresponding frequency distribution, which is a specific sampling distribution dependent on the size of the sample and variability of data.

BOX 11-1

The Central Limit Theorem

The relationship between a population mean and its sampling distribution is known as the Central Limit Theorem. It essentially provides a method to construct a sampling distribution of the population mean. It provides a way to analyze data so that we can test the null hypothesis.

The Central Limit Theorem states:

1. A distribution of sample means from a population will approach the normal distribution, even if the original data were not normally distributed.
2. The mean value of all the possible sample means, $\bar{X}_{\bar{x}}$, will equal the mean of the original population, μ.
3. The standard error of the mean ($SE_{\bar{x}}$) depends on the original standard deviation and size of the sample. The standard error will be much smaller than the sample standard deviation. A larger sample size will result in an even smaller standard error and draw the curve in tighter.

The standard error of the mean ($SE_{\bar{x}}$) can be calculated from the standard deviation and the sample size. It is not necessary to know this, but for those interested, the formula for the standard error of the mean is:

$$SE_{\bar{x}} = \frac{S}{\sqrt{n}}$$

The fact that multiple samples will give different estimates of μ based on their innate variability is referred to as sampling error. It is not really an error; it is a function of the differences we would see if we were to study multiple samples of the same size, as in Figure 11-3. The frequency distribution of all possible sample means has a special application. If we take just one sample and find the mean and standard deviation, we can use the sample data as evidence to support or reject the null hypothesis based on results we would expect from the sampling distribution.

Because we use sample statistics to estimate population parameters, there is a margin of error on either side of the test statistic. This is the confidence interval, which is now a familiar concept:

- *The confidence interval is the estimate of the population parameter ± a margin of error.*

SHOPPING FOR THE RIGHT SAMPLING DISTRIBUTION

Sampling distributions come in a variety of shapes and sizes. The correct one to use depends on the type of test being done. You can depend on your statistician to pick the correct test and type of sampling distribution. I have included a brief discussion here on this topic for those who are interested in knowing about the more common ones. All you really need to understand is that they are all used to plot the test statistic and determine the probability that we would get the result we did if it were due to a chance occurrence.

Many sampling distributions are normal distributions, as we saw in the Z test in Chapter 9. We use the Z statistic when the population standard deviation, μ, is known. A t statistic is used to compare means between groups when μ is not known, which is frequently the case. This statistic is useful when we are comparing two pathways and the outcome variable is measured on an interval scale. It uses t-distributions, which are bell-shaped and analogous to the Z distribution, but there is a specific distribution for each sample size.

When we want to compare proportions in two or more groups, we generate a chi-square statistic. We interpret it on a chi-square distribution, which has a skewed shape. This is especially useful with categorical data. For instance, the chi-square test can be used to compare the proportions of different religions in the various U.S. states, as was discussed in Chapter 4.

Two other distributions with statistical importance are the binomial and Poisson distributions. These are used in specific situations that involve discrete variables. They are briefly mentioned here so you may become familiar with the situations in which they apply.

The binomial distribution is used when the outcome is one of two possible values, such as yes or no, cure or no cure, or success or failure. The distributions illustrate the probability of observing a certain number of successes in a given number of trials, akin to flipping a coin. If you flipped a coin 10 times, you would expect about 5 heads, mathematically denoted as 50% success. The binomial equations can tell us the probability of seeing 2, 1, or even 0 heads (yes, it could happen. The chances are 0.001, or one out of a thousand!). In the same way, you could determine the expected outcome of an event with a 20% chance of success over many trials, and see whether your observation deviated significantly from what you would expect based on chance alone.

The Poisson distribution is used when evaluating a small number of discrete entities evenly dispersed over a large quantity of some medium, such as particles dispersed in air or water. It is also used when observing discrete occurrences over time, such as random genetic mutations. In each case, the population parameter must be known, such as the expected number of entities in a given amount of medium, or expected events over time. This distribution is used to assess whether the data deviates from the expected counts.

Each type of distribution (e.g., normal, binomial, Poisson, or chi-square) has its own distinctive shape. The specifics of the curve, such as height, spread, and slope, will depend on the sample size, n. These details have a greater effect in the shape of the distribution when n is relatively small. As n increases, the effects are subtler. These differences in the shape of the curve do not alter the total area under it; this will always be equal to 1.

How do we deal with so many possible curves when trying to interpret a test statistic? Actually, there are published tables for each type of distribution. For instance, if we have a chi-square value we consult a chi-square table, which can be found in the appendix of most statistics textbooks. The table is compiled from several chi-square distributions for different sample sizes. The value of chi-square will have a corresponding area under the curve that it delineates. The Z score is a type of test statistic which is used when comparing values to a population with a known standard deviation. The table lists the area on either side of a standardized Z score. In this case, it is not necessary to correct for the sample size.

THE CRITICAL VALUE

When a statistician analyzes the data and plugs the values into the appropriate formula, a test statistic results. S/he then consults the corresponding table of values to get an idea of how likely it is that this result would have happened by chance alone. (Many computer programs have these tables stored and will apply the result to the appropriate distribution. A corresponding *p* value will be reported.) We know that any value of a test statistic is possible, but some are more likely than others to happen by chance variation of samples. We decide in advance at which point we are willing to take the risk of a Type I error and declare a true treatment difference, or significant difference. This is called the *significance level*, and is often set at $\alpha = 0.05$.

The value of the *test statistic* that defines this point at which we are willing to say that the result is too unlikely to have happened by chance is called the *critical value*. We may be making a Type I error by rejecting the null hypothesis when it is indeed true, but we are willing to accept that small risk. If our test statistic goes beyond this critical value, then the chance of this result from a random occurrence is very unlikely.

- *The critical value is the value of the test statistic that delineates the specified significance level, which is often 5%.*

PROBABILITY AND INFERENCE

Recall that the probability of an event or outcome is expressed as a fraction between 0 and 1. In the case of sampling distributions, all outcomes from all the possible samples of a uniform size have been accounted for. Basic logic states that when all possible outcomes are considered, the probability is 1 that at least one of these outcomes will occur. The total area below any distribution curve can be considered equal to 1. Any portion of this area is a fraction between 0 and 1. This area can be translated directly into probability. For a segment of a curve that encompasses 50% of the area, the probability is 0.5 that one of these events will occur. For a segment of less than 5%, there is a probability of less than 0.05 that one of these events will occur. When $p < 0.05$, we say there is a less than 5% chance that a test statistic at least as extreme as this would have occurred by chance alone.

- *The area of a segment of the sampling distribution is directly proportional to probability.*

The area under a portion of a curve can be found using calculus methods. This can be quite tedious for many folks so, as we have seen, tables have been published that report the area of segments of these distributions. An important point to be made is that this whole process only works under the assumption that the sample is chosen following the rules of random selection. This ensures that the test statistic behaves predictably. If random selection has been breached, then the logic is flawed and the process is invalid. There are actually ways to mathematically correct for samples that are "less than random." For instance, many surveys are done in clusters rather than following a strict random selection process. It is beyond the scope of this book to discuss when or how this mathematical correction is done, but be aware that the results will still be valid as long as this transgression is recognized and accounted for.

If we are investigating an association between variables, we use a different test but we still interpret it in an analogous way. If there were no true link between the value of one variable and the other, the pairs of numbers would not match. There would be a *predictably random* pattern in the pairs of values. If a stronger pattern emerges that seems unlikely if there were no true link, we reject the null hypothesis of no association and we declare the alternative hypothesis to be true.

KEY POINTS

- The sample data are used to calculate an overall group response.
- If we studied multiple samples from the same population, we would get different results.
- Each result has a frequency with which it would occur if all possible sample combinations of the same size were studied.
- If we were to plot the frequency of a certain result that we would get if we could study all the possible samples, we see a pattern called the sampling distribution.
- The sampling distribution can follow a normal distribution or it can take another shape, depending on the type of data and the question asked.
- Inferential statistics allows us to answer "How likely is it that we would observe this result if the null hypothesis were correct?"
- Samples act in a predictable fashion. The sampling distribution is a collection of expected values.
- We plug the sample data into an equation which results in a test statistic. The particular equation depends on the type of variable(s) and the question being asked.
- The test statistic is a single number that assesses the compatibility of the data with the null hypothesis. We plot the test statistic on its corresponding distribution to see the likelihood, or probability p, that we would get this result if the null hypothesis were true.
- If the result is too improbable, we reject the null hypothesis of no treatment difference, or no relationship between variables, and declare the alternative hypothesis to be true.

REFERENCES

1. Hooke, R. 1983. *How to tell the liars from the statisticians.* New York: Marcel Dekker, Inc.
2. Glantz, S. A. 1992. *Primer of biostatistics*, 3rd ed. New York: McGraw-Hill, p. 23.
3. Glantz, S. A. 1992. *Primer of biostatistics*, 3rd ed. New York: McGraw-Hill, p. 28.

REVIEW QUESTIONS

1. The _____ _____ is a frequency distribution of all possible test statistics that could result from same size samples.

2. The probability of obtaining a particular test statistic from a sample correlates with the _____ of the curve at that point.

3. _____ _____ that occur at the ends of the distribution are less likely to occur by chance.

4. The value of the test statistic that defines the point at which we are willing to reject the null hypothesis is the _____ _____.

5. The critical value often delineates a probability of _____ that the result could happen by chance if the null hypothesis is correct.

ANSWERS TO REVIEW QUESTIONS

1. sampling distribution

2. height

3. Test statistics

4. critical value

5. 0.05 or 5%

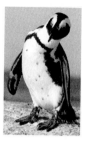

CHAPTER 12

Types of Statistical Tests

Statistics is the essence of the scientific method—it is used across all major disciplines.

—D. B. Owen and Nancy R. Mann[1]

All statistical tests are designed to answer the question of whether or not to reject the null hypothesis. The nuance of the null hypothesis changes slightly in each different application, but overall it states that the variability that is seen in the sample data is due to random variation. Remember that random variation follows an expected pattern that is outlined by the sampling distribution. If the data are very unlikely to occur due to chance, we reject the null hypothesis and adopt the alternative hypothesis. This logic is consistent in each statistical test.

There are many types of statistical tests that can be done, depending on the type of variables and the question being asked. This chapter will discuss a few of the more commonly used tests. The formulas have not been included here because they are not fundamental to understanding the common process used when we do hypothesis testing. As you know, the *p* value is interpreted the same way no matter what type of test is used.

CHI-SQUARE

This frequently used test can tell us whether there is a difference in the proportion of a categorical variable that deviates from what would be expected if the variable were evenly distributed among the different groups, as the null hypothesis would state. It goes by the "goodness-of-fit" test because it assesses whether or not the observed data fit an expected pattern if the null hypothesis is correct. It also is used to check for trends.

The formula for the chi-square statistic χ^2 is a sum of the differences in each cell from what is observed versus what would be expected if the null hypothesis were true. It can be extremely complicated as the number of cells increases. The statistic may be large—into the double or even triple digits. The larger the statistic, the less likely that the null is true and that you would get these results in a random sample. Figure 12-1 is an example of a simple dataset which is used to answer the question: "Is there a significant difference between males and females with respect to their likelihood of being in poverty?"

Only the one-tail test can be done with the chi-square statistic. Also, if there are more than two groups and we get a statistically significant result, we can only say that as least *one* of the groups is significantly different from the rest. To make comparisons among all the groups requires additional statistical methods.

THE STUDENT'S *T*-TEST

This test can be used to see whether there is a difference between sample means in two groups if the variables are continuous. It is used to test for a significant difference due to treatment, or to see whether there has been a change in one group before and after treatment.

The sample is divided into two groups—one that gets an intervention, for example, and one that does not. If the intervention has no effect, then the means of the outcome variable in the two groups would not differ appreciably. When one sample mean is subtracted from the other, the difference is close to zero. The null hypothesis states that the means of the outcome variables in the two groups will be the same and that the treatment difference is zero.

The *t* statistic is analogous to the *Z* statistic and, as the sample gets larger, the distribution for *t* resembles the *Z* distribution. We can perform a two-tailed test with these distributions, so we can test for a difference in either direction.

CORRELATION

In the real world, we observe that certain variables seem to be connected or related. For instance, hair color and eye color tend to be linked. Variables that are linked together are said to *correlate*. One does not necessarily cause the other but they tend to occur together. When the value of one is plotted against another for a given subject, a relationship is visibly apparent as the points tend to cluster along a straight line. The strength of the correlation is expressed as a number called the *Pearson correlation coefficient* (expressed as *r*).

In the sample given below, there are 300 females and 200 males. Is there a significant difference between males and females in their likelihood of being in poverty?

	Females	Males	Total
In poverty	150 (cell a)	50 (cell b)	200
Out of poverty	150 (cell c)	150 (cell d)	300
Total	300	200	500

FIGURE 12-1 If there were no difference between males and females with respect to their likelihood of being poor, the proportion of males and females in poverty should not be significantly different. See www.brynmawr.edu/Acads/GSSW/Vartanian/Handouts/ChiSqu.Examples 2007 for full explanation.

The Pearson correlation coefficient can vary between −1 and 1. A tighter relationship with less scatter will have a Pearson correlation coefficient closer to either −1 or 1. When $r = 1$, there is a perfect correlation (which never happens in nature!). When plotting the data, this results in a perfectly straight line with a positive slope. When $r = -1$, a perfectly straight line with a downward slope results; the variables have a negative correlation. This means the presence of a higher value of one variable is linked to a lower value of the other. When $r = 0$, there is absolutely no correlation and the points are randomly dispersed. The null hypothesis states that $r = 0$.

When the variables have a direct linear relationship, an incremental increase in one affects the other. The slope of the line accounts for the degree of impact. The tightness of the points around this line is reflected in a higher (positive or negative) value of r. Some variables may be linked through a nonlinear relationship. A curved line may be the best fit for the paired variables, which means the value of one is linked to a higher function of the other. This does not affect the interpretation of the Pearson correlation coefficient or its corresponding p value. Figure 12-2 shows examples of associations between two variables.

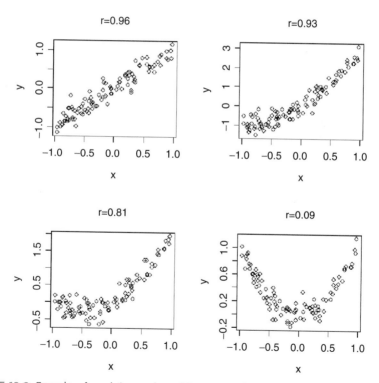

FIGURE 12-2 Examples of correlation graphs and Pearson correlation coefficient for several theoretical associations between the variables x and y. From http://math.uprm.edu/~wrolke/esma3103/graphs/correlationfig4.png August 2007.

REGRESSION

Correlation measures the strength and direction of two linked variables. Regression, on the other hand, measures the strength of an association when one variable helps to explain or predict the other. Regression equations are modeled after the familiar algebraic equation for a straight line, $y = bx + a$, which was discussed in Chapter 2, Mathematical Principles. If we were to solve for y (the response variable) for a given value of x (the explanatory variable), we would have an exact answer. But biostatistics starts with values of x and y for every subject and attempts to find the best equation or model to explain the relationship. The result is a line that best fits the data, which is essentially the line with the least amount of deviation of the points.

The null hypothesis states that there is no significant relationship between the variables and that the slope $b = 0$. A significant result would mean that it is likely that there is a relationship between the values of x and y that is not explained by chance alone. Regression is a powerful tool because it can test for the association between many explanatory variables and the outcome, and can weigh the independent effect of each one. It can also test for nonlinear relationships between explanatory and response variables. Multiple regression is used when the outcome variable is continuous, whereas logistic regression is used for dichotomous outcome variables.

ANALYSIS OF VARIANCE (ANOVA)

This statistical test, like the t-test, deals with the differences between means but, unlike the t-test, it has the ability to compare multiple groups. It does this by comparing the variability within each group to the variability within the entire sample. There are some underlying assumptions in ANOVA, namely, that the values are normally distributed and that the variances of the groups are similar. The null hypothesis states that all the group *means* are equal. If this is true, the *variances* of the group means should not be significantly different from that of the entire sample. The F-test is the significance test that compares the variances.

ANOVA is a very useful tool since it can assess the effects of multiple, independent variables simultaneously. It can also detect an interaction, that is, whether the effect of a particular variable is altered by the presence of a third variable.

MANN–WHITNEY TEST

Variables that are not normally distributed are tested for significance by a different measure of central tendency other than the population means. These are referred to as *nonparametric* tests.

The Mann–Whitney test ranks each individual score in the sample and then compares the sums of ranks between the groups. The null hypothesis states that the sums of the rank data should be the same because there should be no tendency for ranks to be higher or lower if the groups are the same. If the groups are different, then the rank data of the groups will diverge. The Wilcoxon test is a similar test using paired subjects. The Kruskal–Wallis test is similar to ANOVA but is used with ranked data. It compares multiple groups to see whether the sums of ranks is similar, as the null hypothesis would state.

SPEARMAN'S CORRELATION TEST

Ranked data can also be tested for correlation, in which case the Spearman correlation coefficient can be calculated and tested against the null hypothesis of no correlation for the ranked data, which assumes that an increase in rank in one variable for a subject is not associated with an increase or decrease in the other. It is interpreted in the same way as the Pearson correlation coefficient. This is used when the data are non-normal or when they have been recorded by rank.

KEY POINTS

- The chi-square test checks for differences in the proportion of a variable among the groups.
- When two variables are linked for each subject, they are said to correlate.
- Regression checks for the independent effect of several explanatory variables on the outcome response variable.
- ANOVA is a test that checks for differences in several group means by examining the variances of each group and comparing them to the variance of the sample.
- Rank data are assessed by nonparametric tests that do not assume a normal distribution of the variable.

REFERENCE

1. Owen, D. B. and N. R. Mann (Series Editors) in: Hooke, R. 1983. *How to tell the liars from the statisticians.* New York: Marcel Dekker, Inc.

RECOMMEND READINGS

Howell, D. C. 1999. *Fundamental statistics for the behavioral sciences*, 4th ed. Pacific Grove, CA: Brooks/Cole Publishing Co.
Moore D. S. and G. P. McCabe. 1999. *Introduction to the practice of statistics*, 3rd ed. New York: W. H. Freeman and Co.
www.statsoft.com/textbook 2005
www.udel.edu/~mcdonald 2005

R E V I E W   Q U E S T I O N S

1. _____implies an association between two variables, but not cause and effect.

2. Regression models measure the _____ of the effect of one variable on the outcome.

3. Regression methods can also check for the independent effect of several _____ on the outcome.

4. For non-normal data, _____ tests are used that look at other measures, such as rank instead of sample means.

5. Chi-square tests check for differences in the _____ of a variable in the different groups.

ANSWERS TO REVIEW QUESTIONS

1. Correlation

2. strength

3. variables

4. nonparametric

5. proportion

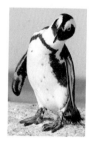

CHAPTER **13**

Properties of Confidence Intervals

Statistical inference ... provides a statement, expressed in the language of probability, of how much confidence we can place in our conclusions.

—David S. Moore and George P. McCabe[1]

We know that we use sample statistics to estimate the unknown population parameter, such as the population mean, μ. This parameter is very real and does not vary, but we cannot measure it—we can only estimate it. How accurate is our estimate? We can answer that question by using confidence intervals, a concept that was introduced by the distinguished Polish statistician Jerzy Neyman in 1937. Confidence intervals are like umbrellas that attempt to encompass the population parameter we are estimating.

When we are under a big umbrella, we feel protected and safe. That is the same feeling we get with a big confidence interval that contains a wide range of values. It is very likely to contain the population parameter we are trying to estimate. Of course, a wide range of values has limited usefulness for pinning down the parameter. We are not sure where that parameter lies within the interval, but we are confident that the interval is very likely to contain it. That is the trade-off for feeling secure in our estimate. If we want 99% confidence, the interval will be larger than if we accept 90% confidence. As we have seen, it is quite common to accept a 95% confidence interval. That means if the study were repeatedly done with the same-sized sample, 95% of the time our confidence interval would include the true population parameter.

For instance, if we are measuring the birth weights of infants born to mothers who smoke, we may take a random sample of 25 infants, weigh them at birth, and average the weights. We are trying to estimate the true population mean weight of all infants born to smoking mothers. We assume the weights are normally distributed. Say we obtained a sample mean of 6 lbs, with a standard deviation of 1 lb (fictitious data). Using the Central Limit Theorem, we calculate a standard error of the sampling distribution to be 0.2 lb. To calculate the confidence interval, the formula is:

Estimate ± margin of error.

113

The estimate refers to the sample statistic that is generated as a result of the data analysis. In this case, it is the sample mean. The margin of error is dependent on three things:

1. The standard deviation of the sample data.
2. The sample size.
3. The confidence we desire, which is usually 95%.

The exact formula will vary depending on the type of data we have, but these three values contribute to the range of values that is obtained regardless of the specific formula. Those who wish to view these formulas are referred to a standard statistics textbook.

The calculated confidence interval for the above data came out to be:

$$6 \pm 0.40 \text{ lb, or } 5.60 \text{ to } 6.40 \text{ lbs at the } 95\% \text{ confidence level.}$$

This interval has a 95% probability of including μ. We are 95% *confident* that our confidence interval contains μ. (This is not the same as stating that μ has a 95% chance of being within these limits. Since μ is constant, it either is or is not within these limits. It is a subtle but valid point.) If we repeated the experiment multiple times with same-sized random samples, the confidence intervals would bounce around the invisible μ. Over repeated sampling, 95% of the confidence levels would capture μ. Figure 4-1 in Chapter 4 represents the sample statistic and 95% confidence intervals of several samples of the same size. Note that the confidence intervals contain ranges of slightly different lengths. This is because each sample will have a different standard deviation, which is one of the factors that affect the size of the confidence interval.

One way to reduce the breadth of the interval is to reduce the significance level for the same size sample. If we are willing to miss the true parameter 10% of the time instead of 5% of the time, we can reduce the confidence level to 90%. This results in a smaller confidence interval of:

$$6 \pm 0.34 \text{ lb, or } 5.66 \text{ to } 6.34 \text{ lbs.}$$

Our interval has narrowed, but at the expense of increased probability of missing μ.

To increase our chances of capturing μ, we can increase the confidence interval to 99%. The result is:

$$6 \pm 0.56 \text{ lb, or } 5.44 \text{ to } 6.56 \text{ lbs.}$$

Figure 13-1 illustrates how changing the requirements of the confidence interval changes the margin of error and results in changing the probability of capturing μ.

Larger sample sizes generally give more accurate results. We are better able to estimate the true population parameter if we have more data. An increase in sample size, therefore, will also narrow the confidence interval. Figure 13-2 shows three different sample sizes taken from a population of infants born to mothers who smoke. The largest sample size has the smallest confidence interval. However, very large sample sizes will have less effect on the range of the confidence interval.

The interval will also be tighter if there is less deviation or scatter of the values in the sample. This is not something that can be manipulated, such as sample size; it is

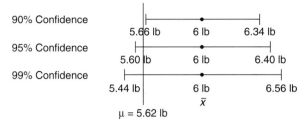

FIGURE 13-1 Confidence intervals for birth weights of infants born to mothers who smoke (fictitious data). If μ is 5.62 lbs, our estimate of 6 lbs captured it at the 95% confidence interval but missed it at the 90% confidence interval. Although intervals at lower limits of confidence are narrower, they run an increased risk of missing the true population parameter.

a characteristic of the population under study. The exact formulas for confidence intervals take standard deviation, sample size, and confidence level into account. In summary, there are three reasons why a confidence interval will be narrower:

- Large sample size.
- Small standard deviation of sample data.
- Relatively low confidence level.

The confidence interval is a way of conveying the relative laxity or tightness of the sampling distribution. Wider intervals are less useful at pinpointing μ than are more compact intervals. In general, narrower intervals are more reassuring and tell us the data are more reliable in their estimate of the parameter.

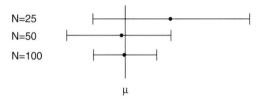

FIGURE 13-2 Sample means and confidence intervals that attempt to capture the true population parameter μ at 95% confidence when the sample sizes are different. The largest sample has the narrowest interval.

KEY POINTS

- The confidence interval attempts to capture the population parameter.
- The range of the interval depends on three things: the standard deviation of the data, the sample size, and the confidence level we desire (usually 95%).
- We can narrow the confidence interval by decreasing the confidence level.
- A more effective way to narrow the interval is to increase the size of the sample.
- Very large sample sizes will have diminishing returns on the effect of the range of the confidence interval.

REFERENCE

1. Moore, D. S. and G. P. McCabe. 1999. *Introduction to the Practice of Statistics*, 3rd Ed. New York: W. H. Freeman and Co.

R E V I E W   Q U E S T I O N S

1. The confidence interval is the estimate of the parameter plus or minus the _____ __ _____.

2. Narrower _____ _____ are more useful than wide ranges of numbers.

3. The range of the confidence interval depends on the _____ _____ of the data, sample _____, and the _____ _____ we desire.

4. One way to decrease the margin of error in our estimation of the parameter is to _____.

A N S W E R S   T O   R E V I E W   Q U E S T I O N S

1. margin of error

2. confidence intervals

3. standard deviation, size, confidence level

4. increase the sample size

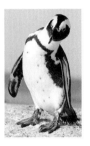

CHAPTER 14

Power

People who play the horses wouldn't think of ignoring the fact that even the greatest horse sometimes loses, but we frequently ignore the fact that even the best experiments sometimes produce no significant difference.

—*David C. Howell*[1]

Throughout our study of biostatistics, we have encountered the concept that in any experiment there is a chance of arriving at the wrong conclusion. We are quite comfortable with the fact that our data may lead us to an incorrect inference. We even have names for the types of errors we could make. However, as long as the chance of error is slim (such as less than 5%), we are willing to accept the risk.

We have carefully considered the possibility of making a Type I error. This is the situation where the data do not support the null hypothesis and, even though there is no true treatment effect or relationship between variables, we have "determined" that there is. We have rejected the null hypothesis of no effect and have erroneously declared that the alternative hypothesis is true. We have not done this intentionally; we are acting on the chance that the data may infrequently lead us astray.

The graphical way to show how we could make an error like this is illustrated in Figure 14-1 by a normally distributed sampling distribution of a sample statistic. If we truly have no treatment effect, then the null hypothesis is true and our test statistic (even though unlikely to occur) did indeed happen. It was our bad luck to get a sample that prompted us to reject the null hypothesis. If this did happen, we would likely be set straight in the future. The results observed in subsequent experiments would not support these original findings, or the results when the treatment is applied in the community would not be as positive.

If we were concerned with the possibility of making a Type I error, we could set our α level very low, say 0.01, to minimize this possibility. However, when we do this, we are less likely to detect a true treatment difference if one does indeed exist. A test with that small a level of α is not very useful because it almost never rejects H_0. When we decrease the chance of a Type I error, we increase the chance of a Type II error, which would incorrectly declare *no* treatment effect. We would like a test to minimize the margin of error to avoid making a Type I error, but we also want a test that has the ability to detect a true treatment difference.

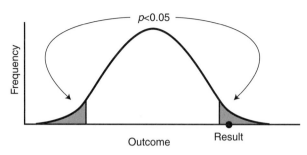

FIGURE 14-1 Sampling distribution of sample means when H_0 is true. This unlikely result caused us to reject the null hypothesis of no treatment effect, even though it was true. $\alpha = 0.05$, using a two-tailed test. This is a Type I error. This could happen, on the average, 1 time out of 20.

If the treatment really did make a difference, then there are really two different sampling distributions—one for the control group and one for the treatment or alternative group. This is an important concept that explains the essence of statistical tests. The reason we get a difference in results (even accounting for variability among the groups) is that the distributions of the outcome variable are different for each group now that one of them has been changed due to the intervention. This is a complex mathematical way of saying, quite simply, that there is a true difference in outcome due to the intervention.

When we compare two groups that have been exposed to an intervention, we look at the difference in means of the outcome variable of the two groups. This is expressed as δ. The null hypothesis would state the groups are the same, and $\delta = 0$. If the treatment has an effect on the outcome, the means of these groups will be more spread out, as in Figure 14-2. The sample statistic (and resulting test statistic) that we get is not likely to be compatible with the results we would get if the null hypothesis were true.

Sometimes the treatment works but it is more subtle. The difference between the outcomes in the groups will not be as apparent and the curves will have more overlap, as in Figure 14-3. Because the difference is smaller, it is easier to miss a true difference even if one exists because our results could still be well within what we would expect for no treatment difference.

If our test statistic fell within the range of values that was consistent with H_0, we would incorrectly assume there was no treatment effect. We do not reject H_0 and we state that the data support no treatment effect, but we are incorrect in doing so. This is a Type II error. It becomes more of a problem when there is only a small difference in the outcome being measured.

Type II errors are reported as though there were no treatment effect, if they are reported at all. These results may end up on a dusty shelf without enjoying the notoriety of their sister studies that were able to show significant results. It is in the best interest of the researcher and the subjects to design a study that would minimize the chance of a Type II error. This would enhance the power of a study, which is the probability of correctly rejecting a false H_0. It is customary to accept this probability at 80%.

- *Power is the probability of correctly rejecting H_0 when a particular alternative value of the parameter is true.*

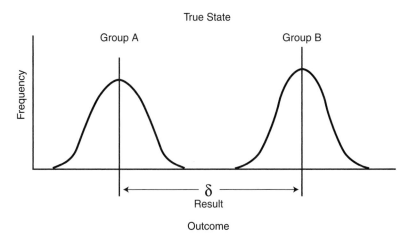

FIGURE 14-2 In a true treatment effect, the difference in observed outcome is largely due to the effect of the intervention rather than random variability of the results. The result is more compatible with the alternative hypothesis than with the null. We have correctly rejected the null hypothesis and declared a true treatment effect.

If we wanted to enhance the power of a study, how would we do this? If we change the significance level so that $\alpha = 0.1$, we are more likely to declare a significant difference and reject H_0 because our test statistic may now fall outside the more lenient critical value. However, that might inadvertently result in a Type I error. We would be more likely to reject H_0 but we have increased the possibility of being wrong to 1 out of 10 times instead of 1 out of 20. We had better stick with the conventional 95% significance.

To increase power, we effectively want to separate the curves that represent the outcomes. We know that a distribution will be narrower if there is a smaller standard deviation or standard error, but that is not something that we can control.

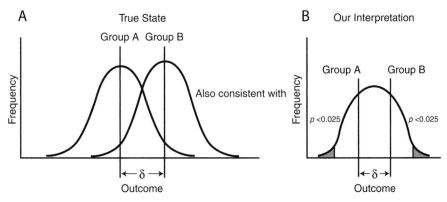

FIGURE 14-3 There is a true but subtle treatment effect. The means of the outcome variable are different but close in value. We cannot reject the null hypothesis at the 5% significance level. This is a Type II error.

How about sample size? It is true that a larger sample size will result in a narrower sampling distribution, and this is a factor that we *can* control. In fact, there are equations to calculate the sample size needed to find a significant effect (if there is one) at a given level of power. The calculation also accounts for a level of significance (often 5%), a value for δ, and the standard deviation or standard error. These can be estimated by using data from similar published studies or by doing a smaller pilot study.

Figure 14-4 illustrates what happens to the sampling distributions as the power of a study is increased for a particular value of δ. Even though the parameter δ remains

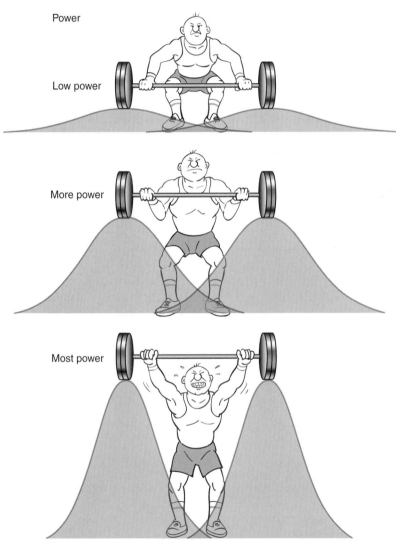

FIGURE 14-4 When there is a true treatment difference, H_0 is not correct, and our ability to correctly state this increases when there is less overlap in the sampling distributions. As power increases, the weight lifter is able to "reach higher" to effectively isolate the curves to minimize the possibility of a Type II error.

the same, it is more likely to be declared a significant difference when there is less overlap of the curves. This can be accomplished by increasing sample size. The test statistic thus becomes a more reliable indicator of the true existence of a significant difference in the outcomes.

We can calculate the number of subjects we will need to enroll by considering the power of the significance test, the value of α, the value of δ, and the standard deviation. It is like estimating the amount of food needed for a company picnic. We can estimate the amount we need based on how much food was consumed in prior years and how many people we expect to show up. It is always better to have too much food, just as it is always safe to sign up a few extra subjects. We take into account the fact that our estimated standard error may be slightly inaccurate and that some subjects will drop out before the study ends.

BOX 14-1

Sample size calculations vary depending on the type of analysis. The general formula is:

$$N = \left[\frac{(z' + z'')\sigma}{\mu_2 - \mu_1} \right]^2$$

Where $(z' + z'')$ is a function of desired power and significance level which can be obtained from a table. We see that sample size, in order to reduce a Type II error, can be determined from power, significance level, the estimated standard deviation, and the detectable effect size which is reflected in the denominator. There are several web sites that do the calculation when the appropriate numbers are filled in.

For instance, if we were to perform an experiment with 25 subjects, for a difference of effect size of 5 on a data set with a normal distribution, mean of 50 and standard deviation of 15, at the 0.05 significance level, the power of the test would be 0.38. This means that when H_0 is truly false, and there is a true treatment effect, a significant difference will be detected only 38% of the time. Using sample size calculations, the power can be increased to 0.80 by increasing sample size to 71 subjects.

KEY POINTS

- We are comfortable with the fact that the data could lead us to reject H_0 even when it is true. This Type I error happens 5% of the time if we accept the standard 0.05 significance level.
- When there is a true treatment effect and we do not reject H_0, we are making a Type II error.
- Power is the probability of correctly rejecting H_0 when it is false.
- One way to increase power is to increase the size of the sample.
- A sample size calculation solves for N, the number of subjects needed to minimize the chance of a Type II error.

REFERENCE

1. Howell, D. C. 1999. *Fundamental statistics for the behavioral sciences*, 4th Ed. Pacific Grove, CA: Duxbury Press.

R E V I E W   Q U E S T I O N S

1. The power of a study is its ability to correctly _____ H_0 and realize that a true treatment effect exists.

2. Higher power will result from a _____ sample size, all other things being equal.

3. When we incorrectly _____ ___ _____ H_0, we are making a Type II error.

A N S W E R S   T O   R E V I E W   Q U E S T I O N S

1. reject

2. larger

3. fail to reject

CHAPTER **15**

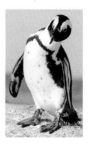

Bias

The science of statistics has made great progress in this century, but progress has been accompanied by a corresponding increase in the misuse of statistics.

—*Robert Hooke*[1]

Bias is a normal human trait. It is the expectation of outcomes in certain scenarios, based on our prior experiences. It molds our behavior by encouraging us to choose situations we find comfortable and predictable. It unconsciously influences our decisions to act in a certain way.

For instance, if you were to attend a banquet it is very likely that you would choose to sit at a table with people you know. You feel comfortable with these people and, from past experience, you subconsciously predict that you will have an enjoyable time. In this way, your decision on where to sit is biased.

Now take the example of a surgeon who is about to perform a redo herniorrhaphy. This is a complex surgical procedure that requires a revision of an original hernia operation. Imagine there are two types of procedures for this operation, and the surgeon is skilled in both. She asks two of her colleagues for their opinion on the better type of procedure. One is a senior surgeon with extensive experience and the other is a junior partner with less experience.

Based on their respective experience levels, the senior surgeon recommends the first procedure, in opposition to the junior surgeon, who recommends the second. The inquiring surgeon is biased (but not to her patient's detriment) in that she will most likely trust the opinion of the senior surgeon. However, a valid study is available that shows the senior surgeon's preference has a higher rate of complications, all other things being equal. The inquiring surgeon must make a decision in the best interest of her patient but, if she still chooses to perform the senior surgeon's preferred operation, she is letting bias influence her decision and is putting her patient at a potential disadvantage.

Bias is often subconscious and unintentional. However, since people who seek medical care must rely on the decisions of their health care professionals, bias in these situations can result in less favorable outcomes. Even though the layperson's interpretation of bias carries a negative connotation akin to prejudice, bias is not a conscious decision to intentionally provide substandard care. Rather, it is acting within a comfort zone based on prior experience with similar patients. In order to

123

minimize bias in the practice of medicine, we must acknowledge its existence and be willing to accept evidence that may alter the way we think.

Experiments are designed to re-create reality. We take a sample group of subjects and study them under controlled conditions, but we try not to alter the real situation that exists so that any conclusions we draw from our observations are valid and can be applied to the entire population. However, experiments are not real situations; they introduce elements that do not reflect the real situation with 100% accuracy. Bias in research is any influence that acts to make the observed results nonrepresentative of the true effect that is under investigation. Again, bias in research is not intentional but a biased study can result in an erroneous conclusion.

- *Bias in statistics is an influence, possibly unrecognized, that introduces error into the process.*

Certain experimental designs are more subject to bias than others, based on the way data are collected. The randomized, blinded, controlled trial was designed to minimize bias and is therefore given more credence than other trial designs. Besides trial design, bias can affect a research study in other ways. It can occur at any point—from the inception of the idea, throughout the trial process of sample selection and data collection, in the analysis, and even in the realm of publication. Bias in research is more detrimental than individual bias because the publicized results can ultimately influence a large number of practitioners.

The following are some areas where you might identify a source of bias. When we critique the literature, we should recognize the potential sources of bias and understand that they could ultimately have an effect on the conclusions upon which we base our recommendations.

Selection bias, in which the populations in the control and treatment groups differ. This is more prevalent in case-control studies since the cases and controls are selected, not randomized. Prospective, nonrandomized cohort studies are also prone to this, since subjects self-select their pathways and their choices may be reflective of some other trait that distinguishes the groups. In trials where the subjects are randomly assigned, this type of bias is minimized. Selection bias can also influence the trial results when the sample is not randomly selected, because the process of inference using sampling distributions is based on random sampling.

Collection bias, in which data (especially in retrospective studies) may be obtained from sources with less than 100% reliability. For example, death certificates do not always list the cause of death accurately. *Recall bias* is a type of collection bias seen in situations where subjects are asked to recall the exposure they had in the past to certain substances. The subjects may have less than accurate recall of these exposures.

Surveillance bias, in which there are differences in follow-up between the groups being studied or in the methods of measurement of the variables. All types of studies are subject to this, but blinding (where subjects and investigators are unaware of the treatment being given) minimizes this effect.

Statistical bias, in which the results are reported in such a way as to promote the investigators' beliefs. Believe it or not, data can be manipulated to give different results. One way to avoid this is to decide upon the type of data analysis before the study commences.

Publication bias, in which journals might not publish valid studies with negative results, or might choose not to publish studies that may seem unimportant at the time. In contrast, a study by a well-known researcher might be more likely to be accepted for publication than the work of a lesser-known investigator, even though both might have equally valid contributions.

Funding bias, in which a well-known researcher is more likely to obtain grant money than an equally qualified but relatively unknown colleague. This allows for the possibility of the more influential investigators to drive the direction of research. This is not necessarily detrimental to medical knowledge, since these folks are the savviest when it comes to setting up trials and they will often have a productive track record. However, less-experienced investigators might not enjoy equal opportunity to launch their projects. It is also a common practice for pharmaceutical companies to fund research studies. This is a well-known source of potential bias—the drug companies want their new drug to outperform the defending champion drug. This enthusiasm might influence the study design and the reported results. Likewise, an investigator might have a financial interest in the outcome of a trial. It is now common practice for a researcher to provide a disclaimer with regard to his or her potential conflict of interest.

Audience bias, in which readers give more credence to studies done in big research centers. Like some other types of bias, this is not necessarily wrong but it should be recognized. Similar to the surgeon in the above scenario, if a reader is unsure of the validity of the study, the past track record of a source of information can help guide his or her decisions. In addition, studies published in foreign languages (even if translations are available) might be underemphasized in favor of those in the native language.

ACCURACY AND PRECISION

We use samples to estimate a population parameter. If a study has been influenced by bias, we may be off the mark and not realize it. The estimate of the population parameter will not be accurate. Even if the study is repeated because of a flaw in design or execution, the dart will consistently miss the target. This shortcoming is reflected in the accuracy of the study.

The results of a study are also affected by the variability of the data. If a particular variable has a large degree of spread in its values, it will be difficult to pinpoint the population parameter even though the design of the study is unbiased. The result will lack precision, which will be reflected in a wide confidence interval. The accuracy of the estimate will not suffer but we may not be able to rely on the results of a single study. Repeating the study will give a different result but multiple studies will eventually hone in on the target. This can be corrected by larger sample sizes.

Figures 15-1 through 15-4 illustrate how accuracy and precision are important when estimating population parameters. If a study has both accuracy and precision, the estimate will be close to the population parameter and repeated studies will show little variability.

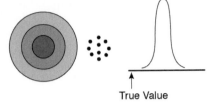

FIGURE 15-1 High precision but low accuracy. *(From Jekel, J. et al. 2001. Epidemiology, biostatistics, and preventive medicine, 2nd ed. Philadelphia: W. B. Saunders Co.)*

True Value

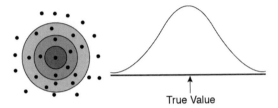

FIGURE 15-2 High accuracy but low precision. *(From Jekel, J. et al. 2001.* Epidemiology, biostatistics, and preventive medicine, *2nd ed. Philadelphia: W. B. Saunders Co.)*

True Value

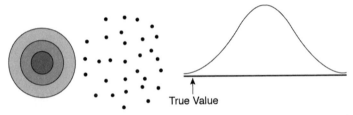

True Value

FIGURE 15-3 Neither accuracy nor precision. *(From Jekel, J. et al. 2001.* Epidemiology, biostatistics, and preventive medicine, *2nd ed. Philadelphia: W. B. Saunders Co.)*

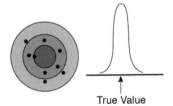

FIGURE 15-4 Both accuracy and precision. *(From Jekel, J. et al. 2001.* Epidemiology, biostatistics, and preventive medicine, *2nd ed. Philadelphia: W. B. Saunders Co.)*

True Value

KEY POINTS

- Bias in the practice of medicine could put the patient at a disadvantage.
- Bias in the medical literature can be highly influential.
- Bias in statistics is an influence, possibly unrecognized, that introduces error into the process.
- Bias can be present at any point of a research project, from its inception to its publication and readership.

- Only by recognizing that bias exists and trying to identify its sources can we minimize it.
- Bias can result in an invalid study in which the results are not accurate but, when repeated, give the same result.
- An imprecise study attempts to approach the mark but, when repeated, is off in another direction. This results from high variability within the samples.
- Accuracy and precision are enhanced by minimizing bias and using proper statistical methods such as random sampling and appropriate sample sizes.

REFERENCE

1. Hooke, R. 1983. *How to tell the liars from the statisticians*. New York: Marcel Dekker, Inc.

REVIEW QUESTIONS

1. Research experiments attempt to study a real situation by using _____ and observing the results.

2. There are many ways that a study may not exactly recreate the real situation. The results are then said to be _____.

3. _____ is not necessarily intentional.

4. Bias affects the _____ of a study.

5. When there is less variability in the sample data, a study will be more precise, and a smaller _____ _____ will be seen.

ANSWERS TO REVIEW QUESTIONS

1. samples

2. biased

3. Bias

4. validity, accuracy

5. confidence interval

CHAPTER **16**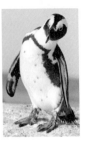

Ethics in Medical Research

Liars, as portrayed on screen and in fiction, are often charming rogues,
while statisticians are always persons of infinite dullness. In real life,
this is not the way you tell one from the other

—*Robert Hooke*[1]

Physicians have always been guided in their profession by a code of ethics. Medical professionals are in the unique position of directing decisions that affect the health and well-being of a trusting public. We make recommendations to folks who have confidence that we will act in their best interest. As early as the fourth century B.C., the Greek physician Hippocrates recognized the importance of the moral responsibility of the physician to the patient. He produced a litany of documents that addressed the basic principle of ethical conduct, "to help and not to harm." The Hippocratic Oath is a product of this era that emphasizes the importance of respecting the ethical rights of the patient. Parts of this oath are still recited by United States medical school graduates as they receive their degree.

There is the potential for a breach of trust in the physician–patient relationship when medical professionals act in a manner that unduly places the patient at risk of harm. One of the most flagrant examples of a deviation from the basic principle of ethical treatment of humans was the barbaric torture that was inflicted upon concentration camp victims by the Nazis during World War II. These heinous actions included hypothermic "experiments" in which subjects were immersed in tanks of ice water and frozen to death. Others were deprived of oxygen and they slowly asphyxiated. Some of the prisoners were deliberately infected with cholera or suffered through grotesque surgeries that involved transplanted organs or sterilization. These appalling interventions were performed on captive victims against their will and under the guise of "medical experimentation."

When these inhumane acts were publicly revealed, there was an international outcry for guidelines to direct the ethical treatment of human subjects in medical experimentation. The Nuremberg Military Tribunal that investigated these war crimes, which ultimately led to the execution of the responsible physicians, compiled a list of conditions outlining acceptable ethics in these circumstances. This came to be known as the Nuremberg Code (see Box 16-1). When it was released in 1947, it introduced the world to the era of modern medical ethics. It provided the basic expectations that should be met when experiments on human subjects are performed.

BOX 16-1

The Nuremberg Code

Permissible Medical Experiments

The great weight of the evidence before us is to the effect that certain types of medical experiments on human beings, when kept within reasonably well-defined bounds, conform to the ethics of the medical profession generally. The protagonists of the practice of human experimentation justify their views on the basis that such experiments yield results for the good of society that are unprocurable by other methods or means of study. All agree, however, that certain basic principles must be observed in order to satisfy moral, ethical and legal concepts:

1. *The voluntary consent of the human subject is absolutely essential. This means that the person involved should have legal capacity to give consent; should be so situated as to be able to exercise free power of choice, without the intervention of any element of force, fraud, deceit, duress, overreaching, or other ulterior form of constraint or coercion; and should have sufficient knowledge and comprehension of the elements of the subject matter involved as to enable him to make an understanding and enlightened decision. This latter element requires that before the acceptance of an affirmative decision by the experimental subject there should be made known to him the nature, duration, and purpose of the experiment; the method and means by which it is to be conducted; all inconveniences and hazards reasonably to be expected; and the effects upon his health or person which may possibly come from his participation in the experiment. The duty and responsibility for ascertaining the quality of the consent rests upon each individual who initiates, directs or engages in the experiment. It is a personal duty and responsibility which may not be delegated to another with impunity.*

2. *The experiment should be such as to yield fruitful results for the good of society, unprocurable by other methods or means of study, and not random and unnecessary in nature.*

3. *The experiment should be so designed and based on the results of animal experimentation and a knowledge of the natural history of the disease or other problem under study that the anticipated results will justify the performance of the experiment.*

4. *The experiment should be so conducted as to avoid all unnecessary physical and mental suffering and injury.*

5. *No experiment should be conducted where there is an a priori reason to believe that death or disabling injury will occur; except, perhaps, in those experiments where the experimental physicians also serve as subjects.*

6. *The degree of risk to be taken should never exceed that determined by the humanitarian importance of the problem to be solved by the experiment.*

7. *Proper preparations should be made and adequate facilities provided to protect the experimental subject against even remote possibilities of injury, disability, or death.*

8. *The experiment should be conducted only by scientifically qualified persons. The highest degree of skill and care should be required through all stages of the experiment of those who conduct or engage in the experiment.*

9. *During the course of the experiment the human subject should be at liberty to bring the experiment to an end if he has reached the physical or mental state where continuation of the experiment seems to him to be impossible.*

Continued

BOX 16-1—cont'd

10. *During the course of the experiment the scientist in charge must be prepared to terminate the experiment at any stage, if he has probable cause to believe, in the exercise of the good faith, superior skill and careful judgment required of him that a continuation of the experiment is likely to result in injury, disability, or death to the experimental subject.*

(From *Trials of War Criminals before the Nuremberg Military Tribunals under Control Council Law No. 10. Nuremberg, October 1946–April 1949. Washington, D.C.: U.S. Government Printing Office, 1949-4953.)*

It echoed the Hippocratic philosophy of "do no harm" and also stressed the importance of informed consent by the subjects.

The international medical community also responded to these atrocities by developing a set of guidelines to ensure that experimentation is carried out under acceptable ethical standards. This document was first released in Helsinki, Finland in 1964 during an international convention of the World Medical Association. It is known as the Declaration of Helsinki, even though it has undergone several revisions since then. It captures many of the principles established by the Nuremberg Code but also distinguishes between therapeutic and nontherapeutic research.

In spite of the formal recognition and endorsement of ethical principles set forth in the Nuremberg Code and Declaration of Helsinki, there have been multiple incidents in the United States in which medical experiments used questionable ethical standards in their design. One of the more notorious was the federal government-sponsored trial of African-American men who had contracted syphilis. The study began in Tuskegee, Alabama in 1932. This was an observational trial that studied more than 600 men to track the physiological effects of syphilis over several decades. Most of these men were poor and illiterate and were kept uninformed of their disease. In addition, they were not offered treatment when it became available a couple of decades after the study began.

The infamous Tuskegee study was one of the catalysts for the development of human experimentation guidelines by the U.S. federal government. In 1974, the National Research Act was passed which established the National Commission for the Protection of Human Subjects of Biomedical and Behavioral Research. Over the next several years, the National Commission issued recommendations that outlined the principles of ethical treatment of human subjects. One of their reports has become the cornerstone of ethical experimentation. It is known as *The Belmont Report*, after the Belmont Conference Center at the Smithsonian Institution where it was conceived. This report promulgates three basic philosophical principles upon which ethical standards should be founded:

1. *Respect for persons* must be maintained. This protects the dignity of the individuals and also includes consideration of their autonomy and their right to make informed decisions on interventions that affect their destiny. This principle emphasizes the need for informed consent. The subjects should understand the potential risks and benefits of participating in a research project. They should be willing participants.

2. *Beneficence* must be considered. This ensures that the health of the individual will take precedence over the research hypothesis. All types of possible harm should be considered and assessed for on a regular basis. The risk of enrollment should be weighed against the potential benefit not only to the individual for his or her participation, but also the benefit to society from the knowledge gained from the study.
3. *Justice* must be upheld. No group should be singled out unfairly to participate for reasons of race, gender, or socioeconomic status. On the other hand, when participation is felt to offer a significant advantage to the individual, all eligible groups should be invited to participate.

The National Commission requires that these fundamental principles be considered in all types of research design and in the execution of experiments. The governing body that upholds these principles is the Institutional Review Board (IRB). This is a local committee specific to each institution; it is made up of a diverse group of medical and nonmedical members, which often includes a cleric or other persons with formal training in medical ethics. The IRB assesses the research on a regular basis, from its inception through its completion. It considers the ethics of the projects with respect to the principles set forth in *The Belmont Report*, and has the right to halt the research if the members feel there is a violation of any of these principles.

When you evaluate the literature, you may run into some gray areas where the question of whether the appropriate ethics have been followed is not crystal clear. Captive audiences, such as prisoners or in-hospital patients, are often targeted as subjects. Even if they are able to give informed consent, is the principle of justice violated? Is it possible they could think they would get better treatment if they participated, and therefore feel pressured to enroll? These examples illustrate why there are ongoing debates over ethical principles and why the collective wisdom of the IRB is crucial. A multitude of opinions on these issues exists and it behooves us to entertain them all.

The ethics of medical experimentation is based on a few sound philosophical principles that capture the wisdom and fairness of the adage "Treat someone as you would want to be treated." When you are faced with an ethical issue that has no easy answer, ask yourself how you would feel if you were the subject. Your response should help guide you in your decision.

KEY POINTS

- The practice of medicine and medical experimentation is guided by a code of ethics.
- Early medical ethicists such as Hippocrates adopted the adage "To help and not to harm." This still underscores the philosophy of modern medical ethics.
- The heinous acts against humans that were performed under the guise of "medical experimentation" during World War II prompted the international Nuremberg Military Tribunal to construct a code of ethics, called the Nuremberg Code, to be followed when medical experiments are performed. It stresses the concept of informed consent, among other things.
- The World Medical Association devised a code of ethics for medical experimentation, called the Declaration of Helsinki. It supports many of the concepts of the Nuremberg Code and also makes a distinction between therapeutic and nontherapeutic research.

- The U.S. government also developed guidelines for human experimentation through the establishment of the National Commission for the Protection of Human Subjects of Biomedical and Behavioral Research. In their *Belmont Report*, they identify three principles of ethical experimentation: Respect for Persons, Beneficence, and Justice.
- The Institutional Review Board (IRB) oversees medical research at the level of the institution to ensure that medical ethics have not been breached.

REFERENCE

1. Hooke, R. 1983. *How to tell the liars from the statisticians.* New York: Marcel Dekker, Inc.

REVIEW QUESTIONS

1. The _____ _____ _____ is a committee at an institution that oversees medical research.

2. The _____ _____ is a code of ethics devised by the Nuremberg Military Tribunal after World War II in response to concentration camp atrocities.

3. The Tuskegee syphilis study did not obtain _____ _____ from its subjects, which prompted the Respect for Persons principle outlined in *The Belmont Report*.

4. The principle of _____ referred to in *The Belmont Report* ensures that no group will be singled out unfairly in medical research.

5. The principle of Beneficence looks after the _____ of the subjects.

ANSWERS TO REVIEW QUESTIONS

1. Institutional Review Board or IRB

2. Nuremberg Code

3. informed consent

4. Justice

5. well-being, health

17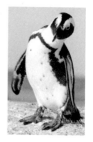

Types of Research Studies

Scientific studies pursue truth. In evaluating a study, the initial consideration is whether the study arrived at this truth successfully.

—D. J. Friedland[1]

Congratulations! You now have the map reading skills necessary to navigate the literature. You will find, as you peruse the journals and other sources of information, that there are several types of studies, each with their own benefits and drawbacks. For instance, the double-blinded, randomized, controlled trial (DBRCT) is considered the gold standard in clinical research. It is purposely designed to minimize potential sources of bias. When it is adequately powered and properly executed, it has both accuracy and precision.

Unfortunately, for various reasons not all trials can be conducted as DBRCTs. Certain criteria have to be met, such as blinding the subjects as to the particular pathway in which they are enrolled. If they are unaware of the treatment to which they are exposed, there will be no subconscious expectations that could potentially influence results. However, certain types of experiments do not lend themselves to blinding. For instance, in studies that compare surgical interventions to medical treatments, neither the subjects nor the researchers can be blinded.

Ethical standards for clinical trials must be met as well. It behooves all researchers to enter into a study with equipoise (discussed in Chapter 10) so that the possibility of either treatment being better, or even potentially harmful, is considered in the analysis. After all, the study is being conducted because we often do not know whether one pathway has an advantage or harbors possible deleterious effects. Participants must be aware of the possibility of harm even though it may be minimal.

Even though the DBRCT has the distinction of producing the most dependable results, many other types of experiments have an important place in clinical literature. Not every trial can be a DBRCT, nor does it need to be. Observational studies, in which people choose their own course and are followed over time, can contribute immensely to the fund of medical knowledge. Most epidemiological studies are done this way, such as the famous Framingham studies that began in 1948.[2] This database recorded, among other things, the lifestyle habits of thousands of individuals and then looked at their subsequent rate of heart disease. This invaluable information led to our current understanding of cardiovascular risk factors.

CASE REPORTS

What prompts an individual to pursue a particular research question? The earliest clue that there could be an association among particular variables may be reported in the simple but intriguing case report. When a clinician sees something out of the ordinary, reporting this in a journal alerts other practitioners to a possible connection. For instance, at a dermatology conference in San Francisco in the early 1980s, a cluster of several cases of homosexual men with an unusual type of skin cancer called Kaposi's sarcoma was reported.[3] Was there a connection between gay men and skin cancer? There most certainly was! This observation led to research that resulted in the identification of the virus that caused a major epidemic of immense ramifications, namely, autoimmune deficiency syndrome (AIDS).

OBSERVATIONAL STUDIES

Once a potential connection between variables has been identified through case reports, observational studies are done that attempt to elucidate the presence and strength of this association. Venn diagrams are a rough way to illustrate observed connections between variables, but they have little scientific validation. Correlation is one way to comment on the strength and direction of the association. The correlation coefficient tells us not only whether there is a significant association, but also the degree of impact of one variable upon another and whether increasing the value of one has a positive or negative association with the other. Correlation does *not* tell us whether one variable *caused* the effect on the other, only that there is a link. When the association is measured at a single point in time (as opposed to the effect over time), this is known as a cross-sectional study.

Keep in mind that two variables may be linked through a third "hidden" variable. This was the case with gay men and Kaposi's sarcoma. The link was eventually identified as the human immunodeficiency virus (HIV). If we were comfortable in assuming that there was no other connection between homosexuality and skin cancer, and did not look further, we would miss this fact. These hidden variables are called *confounders*. They often account for a major portion of the association of other variables through their independent connection with each of them. Do African-American children perform less well in school than Caucasians because of their skin color? Most experts would agree that even though an association between skin color and school performance can be demonstrated, the connection has to do with confounders such as socioeconomic class.

CASE–CONTROL STUDIES

Observational studies can also be done retrospectively. These are known as case–control studies; the outcomes are already known. We take people with the outcome and try to match them in many other respects with healthier counterparts. Then we look back to see if there is a correlation between a particular variable and an adverse outcome. If so, we infer that if we remove that variable we can improve outcome.

For instance, a recent retrospective study looked at a sample from a population of people with heart attacks. All other things being equal, did anemia have an adverse effect on the outcome of mortality? The analysis showed that those with severe anemia fared worse than those with normal blood counts. This supports the use of blood transfusion in those patients with heart attacks who also have severe anemia.[4]

I like to think of case–control studies as people getting off a train at their destination. You greet them at the station named Disease and then look in their suitcases to see what items they have carried with them. Then you go to the Healthy station and see what those individuals have packed. The overall difference in their baggage could account for their destination. For instance, people arriving at the Coronary Artery Disease station will have a greater tendency to pack cigarettes, bacon and eggs, and insulin for their diabetes. They will be more likely to carry the death certificates of parents and siblings who died of heart disease. Those who get off at the Healthy station will have more jogging suits and turkey sandwiches. There will be some overlap of items but you will see a distinct difference in the overall baggage between the two destinations.

Retrospective studies are especially applicable to outcomes that are relatively rare or take a long time to develop. This type of study can be done without waiting for the subjects to develop the disease. One of the limitations of this type of study exists in finding an appropriately matched control group. They need to be similar to the diseased group in all respects (except for the disease and the variable under study). If there is some other difference not accounted for, an unidentified confounding variable could be responsible for the outcome. This could lead to an incorrect conclusion with regard to the other variable under study.

Retrospective studies are also prone to recall bias when they rely on the subjects' memory of exposures to substances. Those with the disease may have more accurate recall of their exposures. On the other hand, the subjects might also overestimate an exposure they believe might have led to the disease. There are some mathematical limitations as well. Calculation of risk involves the development of disease over time, with a common starting point for both disease and disease-free groups. Since we look backward in time, we have no true starting point. This allows us to calculate odds ratios (a measure of association) rather than risk (which reflects a rate).

COHORT STUDIES

When we have the time to wait for the outcome to develop, a prospective study that goes forward in time can be done. Cohort studies start with a group of subjects and measure the relative incidence of disease in those who are exposed to a variable, in comparison to those not exposed. The groups in a prospective study are not necessarily randomized or blinded; they may choose their exposures. The Framingham Study is a good example of a prospective cohort design. Because the exposure preceded the outcome, there is a stronger argument in favor of the exposure causing the disease, although this in itself is insufficient to prove causation. There is a starting point in time, so risk can be calculated. Recall bias is minimized in this design. However, one drawback is the prolonged time and expense these studies require to carry them to completion while waiting for the observed outcome.

RANDOMIZED CONTROLLED TRIALS

This brings us to the poster child for evidence-based medicine, the double-blinded, randomized, controlled trial (DBRCT). There are many potential opportunities for bias to creep into studies, which can ultimately result in an erroneous conclusion. The carefully contrived DBRCT, although not guaranteed to be completely bias-free, has eliminated many types of bias that are woven into other trial designs. This study resembles a prospective cohort study with a few important distinctions.

When subjects agree to participate, they are allocated, through a random process, to one of two or more pathways. If subjects were allowed to choose their pathway, as in an observational study, this would introduce other factors that could account for the outcome. Consider a cancer trial that allows subjects to choose either the Standard of Care Drug or a New Drug. Within this sample of cancer patients, the healthier ones may decide, even subconsciously, to stick with the familiar Standard of Care Drug while the more desperate ones may be willing to take a chance on the new treatment. The point to be made here is that the Standard of Care Drug pathway in this case is destined to have a better outcome, even if it is not a better drug *because the groups going down the two pathways are not the same.* Randomization eliminates the possibility that a treatment could show an erroneous advantage through this type of selection bias. If potential confounders are present (even if they cannot be identified), they should be equally distributed among the groups and thus not contribute to a difference in outcomes.

It is human nature to want to please others. When subjects participate in a trial, there may be a subconscious wish to justify the investigators' efforts and to provide hope to future victims of the same disease. This admirable quality can be deleterious to the process of scientific investigation, however, by producing erroneous conclusions about the true merit of a particular pathway. If subjects or investigators are aware of which pathway is being followed, there may be a tendency to minimize reported symptoms. Through biofeedback mechanisms, it is also possible to psychologically alter measurable processes such as blood pressure. This can result in a falsely inflated benefit in favor of a particular treatment. In a double-blinded trial, this type of bias is eliminated because both the researchers and the subjects are unaware of the treatment that is being given. It is standard for all the groups to receive the same number and type of interventions. For instance, if an oral medicine is being compared to an intravenous one, both groups will get a pill and an infusion. No one knows which is the inert substance. Some placebos go through a rigorous design process so they match their active counterparts in size, color, and consistency.

Even though a well-executed DBRCT is scientifically robust (this is known as having internal validity), one of its drawbacks is the selection process. All the participants are volunteers who are willing and able to contribute to the process of scientific knowledge. They may be better-educated and healthier in general than those who cannot or choose not to participate. The subjects may not be representative of all members of the community who meet the same inclusion and exclusion criteria. The results of a DBRCT, therefore, may not always be externally validated or reproducible to the same degree in the larger community.

The scheme in Figure 17-1 is one way to categorize the type of research that is encountered in the literature. The study design is a key to the type of conclusions that can be drawn as well as the strength of the evidence. Survey studies are not specifically mentioned; most of these may be considered a type of cross-sectional observational study.

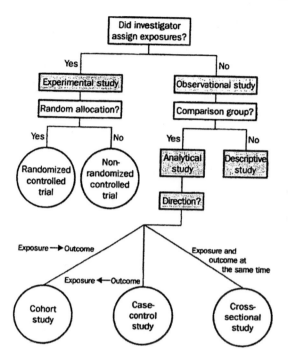

FIGURE 17-1 Algorithm for classification of types of clinical research. *(From Grimes, D. A. et al. 2002. An overview of clinical research: The lay of the land.* Lancet, *359:9300, 58, with permission.)*

FACTORS IN FINAL ANALYSIS

Statisticians need to account for factors that can complicate the final results in a clinical trial. In unblinded trials, some patients cross over into the other treatment arm at the recommendation of their physicians or at their own desire. There are ways to account for this change in the final data analysis, as long as it is recognized. The most reliable method is the "intention to treat" analysis, which assumes that the subjects followed along the original pathway to which they were assigned, no matter what the outcome.

For various reasons, there will also inevitably be dropouts along the way. It is important to take this into consideration when doing a calculation to estimate the appropriate sample size. The reason why subjects leave is not to be underestimated, either. It might be that the intervention had an undesirable side effect so extreme that it became unbearable. It would be important for the investigators to know this. Short of withdrawing from a study, a subject may continue to participate in the trial even though not complying with the treatment recommendations. This can happen for various reasons, including annoying side effects. The more astute studies will have a surveillance system built in, if possible, to check for noncompliance.

There are many instances when the effect of an intervention will be greater in one faction of a sample than another. For instance, lowering serum cholesterol may have a greater effect on outcome in a hypertensive individual than in a normotensive one. It is possible to study an effect on many subsets of the sample by looking at *subgroup analysis*. This is a way to get maximal information from one study design. It is important to have a large enough sample so that all subgroups have an adequate number of subjects for a meaningful subgroup analysis. If one subgroup contains only a few individuals, there may be inadequate power to detect an advantage of the treatment in the subgroup, even if one exists. When studies are in the planning phase, this can be accounted for in the calculation of sample size. Alternatively, the designers can weight the recruitment of subjects so that each subgroup has adequate representation.

REVIEW ARTICLES

There are several situations in which we might need to peruse a collection of articles on a particular subject. For instance, diseases that are prevalent and have a large impact on general health care, such as asthma or congestive heart failure, have been studied extensively. We may encounter several large trials that focus on the same problem. Administrators are often faced with problems in health care policy that affect large populations and consume a major portion of health care resources. Their decisions regarding the organization and delivery of health care should be based on the most recent collective information available.

Review articles have done this work for us. The authors of a review article should inform the reader of the search method used to locate the articles and the decision-making process employed when considering which articles to include in the review. The populations do not need to match exactly since the articles do not combine data; the authors just compile and report the results of several studies with similar interests. Keep in mind that the search may have been conducted a little differently than if you had done it yourself. Delegating the driver's seat to someone else may result in articles with a slightly different profile than those you would have gotten.

Several agencies such as the Cochrane Collaboration (www.cochrane.org/reviews) and the United Health Foundation (www.clinicalevidence.org) perform a formal review service for our convenience. Because they employ a strict scientific method of review, they are called systematic reviews. All articles undergo a rigorous screening process that looks for potential flaws in the design and conclusions. Only the most valid articles are included. This approach enhances the reliability of the review article by minimizing the bias that might be encountered if an individual performed the review.

META-ANALYSIS

The word *meta-analysis* actually means "after the analysis." This type of study integrates the results from several similar prior studies and analyzes the combined information. It is most applicable in the health care administrative arena when assessing the usefulness of interventions to establish broad guidelines and set policy. It can also pinpoint the actual risk of environmental exposures and the development of disease by integrating several epidemiological studies. The purpose of a meta-analysis is to get the answer once and for all, especially in situations where the data seem to support conflicting conclusions.

A properly executed meta-analysis starts out with a research hypothesis, just as in any other type of study. The population is identified based on inclusion and exclusion criteria. Instead of obtaining a sample of individuals from the population, however, the authors do a search of existing research to find studies with similar populations. The data from randomized, controlled trials (RCTs) is generally preferred over observational studies, although there may be limitations on available RCTs which would preclude their exclusive use in the meta-analysis. The data are combined using sophisticated statistical techniques that look at the outcomes of these individual trials and integrate the results. The overall result is known as the *summary measure*. Because these trials will be of different sizes, each result is weighted according to its proportional contribution to the summary measure.

This method can be quite powerful because of the sheer number of subjects that results when studies are combined. We have seen how the power of a study (its ability to detect a treatment difference when one really does exist) is influenced by the number of participants. Increasing the sample size will metaphorically pull apart the bell curves and move our result from a gray zone to a black-and-white conclusion.

Larger sample sizes also provide a more accurate estimate of the population parameter because they have less variability than do smaller samples from the same population. In Chapter 13, we saw mathematically how this happens as the confidence interval gets narrower for larger sample sizes. Meta-analyses also carry the advantage of having less selection bias. Combined studies are more likely to include a representative sample of the population; this will enhance the external validity of the results.

Figure 17-2 shows the results of a meta-analysis that combined data on exposure to environmental tobacco smoke and lung cancer. The summary measure—the overall result of all nine studies—was the odds ratio. It answered the question "In a person who develops lung cancer, what are the odds that he or she was exposed to environmental tobacco smoke?" This graph shows that the summary measure is in accordance with the individual studies and, quite remarkably, how the confidence interval

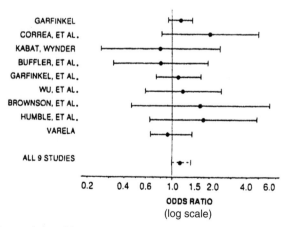

FIGURE 17-2 Meta-analysis: odds ratios and 95% confidence intervals for nine U.S. epidemiologic studies of the hypothesized association between exposure to environmental tobacco smoke and lung cancer. *(From Fleiss, J. L. and A. J. Gross. 1991. Meta-analysis in epidemiology, with special reference to studies of the association between exposure to environmental tobacco smoke and lung cancer: A critique.* J Clin Epidemiol, *44:2, 127–139, with permission.)*

has narrowed when the data were combined. We are 95% certain that we have captured the true parameter odds ratio for the population in this narrow interval.

This type of analysis is appealing because of its scientific strength. It is also relatively inexpensive since the work is done on computers rather than in the field. However, combining data is not as easy as it sounds. This method is hindered by problems unique to the situation created by doing a study on a diverse collection of pre-existing evidence. Every phase must be carefully executed, starting with the literature search. It can be a challenge just to identify and appropriately screen all the pertinent articles. Variation in sample selection may make some studies ineligible since they might not represent the population under study in the meta-analysis. Differences in sample sizes and methodology must also be accounted for when combining studies. Outcome measures might be reported differently from one study to another. In summary, meta-analysis can be a powerful tool but the methodology is tricky and requires sophisticated statistical techniques. The appropriate approach to this complex process is still evolving.[5,6,7]

FUNNEL DIAGRAMS

It is possible that some articles relevant to the research hypothesis of a meta-analysis might not have gotten published because of negative results. One can attempt to identify publication bias in the existing literature by using a funnel diagram. This works on the concept that multiple smaller studies will predictably have greater variability in their results than do larger studies (a variation of the power principle).

If multiple smaller studies tend to report overwhelmingly favorable results, this supports the premise that some smaller studies with less-convincing results might have gotten overlooked due to publication bias. The search should be extended to look for articles in lesser-known journals and for any unpublished results that might be pertinent to the research hypothesis. An example of a funnel diagram is shown in Figure 17-3.

CONDUCTING A LITERATURE SEARCH

When we encounter a situation that requires a perusal of the literature, we have several options. We can do a literature search on our own or we could enlist the help of a librarian. A variety of search mechanisms is available to select and reprint the pertinent articles on a particular topic. Several databases can be accessed through the Internet, including websites of The Cochrane Library (www.cochrane.org) and the Ovid database (www.ovid.com). Another superb search mechanism is U.S. National Library of Medicine's PubMed (www.ncbi.nlm.nih.gov/pubmed). Most search mechanisms look for phrases or words that can be applied to a directory of medical terms. The results you get will depend on the keywords you type in. The search can be cross-referenced with other terms by using Boolean modifiers such as AND, OR, or NOT. You may need to expand your search to be more inclusive if the original results were too skimpy, or narrow it down when you get hundreds of hits. The PubMed web site includes a basic tutorial that will take you through the process.

One method is to initiate the search by looking for review articles on a particular subject. This is more likely to be productive if the condition is prevalent and is a

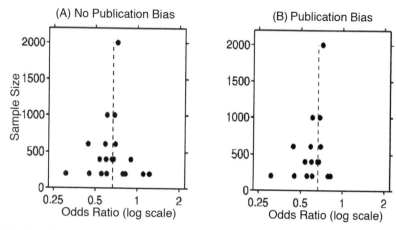

FIGURE 17-3 The results of the studies are plotted against the sample size. A, The graph should assume a funnel-like shape if there is no publication bias; B, Finding only smaller studies with favorable results suggest publication bias. The larger studies will also approximate the true population parameter more accurately than will smaller studies, which will predictably have greater variation in results. *(From Dwamena, B. 2004. Metagraphiti by Stata. 3rd North American Stata Users Group Meeting, August, University of Michigan, with permission.)*

BOX 17-1

How Drugs Get Studied

Before a new drug is released to the public, it has typically been tested on animals for desirable response, dosing, and side effects. From there, it must undergo fastidious testing on humans that usually involves several phases over multiple years.[8,9,10]

Phase I: Clinical Pharmacology and Toxicity

To determine the dose that is best tolerated, with emphasis on pharmacokinetics and side effects of increasing doses. These are often done on healthy volunteers but may also enroll subjects with the disease that will eventually be targeted. These are typically observational studies and the information is used to design Phase II trials.

Phase II: Initial Assessment for Therapeutic Effects

To evaluate effectiveness in a given clinical situation and to continue to assess short-term toxicities along with the best dose–response relationship. A limited number of human subjects are enrolled in these observational studies, usually fewer than 100.

Phase III: Full-Scale Evaluation of Treatment

To compare the results of a new drug to the standard of care with respect to efficacy and toxicity. This is usually a randomized, controlled trial enrolling hundreds of subjects. The drug is administered in the same way as it would be marketed. After this phase, the sponsor may apply for U.S. Food and Drug Administration (FDA) approval.

Phase IV: Continued Observation in the Postmarketing Phase

To check for late side effects and to compare results in the community with subjects in the trials (external versus internal validation).

major health concern. The above resources provide this service, as does the United Health Foundation's Clinical Evidence web site (www.clinicalevidence.com). Another approach is to search for meta-analyses or DBRCTs only, since these are generally more reliable than other types of data. Many search mechanisms have a command that can limit the search to these types of studies. Because many subjects have limited information in these formats, however, the search will need to include observational studies as well. If you have noted an unusual occurrence in a particular patient, you may just want to search for similar case reports. Once the search is completed, the articles can be evaluated for their validity and applicability.

KEY POINTS

- All types of research studies provide important information.
- The type of study that can be done depends on such factors as time frame, ability to blind the subjects, and ethical issues such as informed consent.
- Case reports can identify a previously unrecognized association between variables.
- A case–control study is a type of retrospective observational study that compares the difference in exposure to a substance by starting with individuals who have a disease and comparing the degree of exposure to the same substance in their normal counterparts. An odds ratio can be calculated which reflects the *odds* of a diseased individual having had the exposure compared to a nondiseased individual.
- A cohort study is a prospective observational study. Cases are selected on the basis of exposure and are followed over time. Since we have a starting point, we can measure the risk of disease (the chance of getting the disease over time) in exposed individuals compared to the risk of disease in individuals without the exposure.
- The randomized controlled trial is designed to minimize bias. The potential confounders should be evenly distributed between the groups and should not influence the results.
- A meta-analysis combines the data from multiple studies after they have been done. Its strength lies in the power behind the sheer number of subjects that should result in an accurate estimation of the parameter.
- Funnel diagrams are used to identify publication bias.
- Review articles are compiled from a search of the literature. A systematic review uses a strict scientific design to ensure the inclusion of all pertinent information and to screen for bias.
- Before drugs are released to the public, they must undergo rigorous testing in several consecutive phases to assess efficacy and toxicity.

REFERENCES

1. Friedland, D. J. 1998. *Evidence-based medicine: A framework for clinical practice*. Stanford, CT: Appleton and Lange.
2. Dawber, T. W. 1980. *The Framingham study*. Cambridge, MA: Harvard University Press.
3. http://en.wikipedia.org/wiki/Kaposi's_sarcoma. 2005.
4. Wu, W. C. et al. 2001. Blood transfusion in elderly patients with acute myocardial infarction. *New Engl J Med*, 345:17, 1230.

5. Kjaergard, L. L. et al. 2001. Reported methodologic quality and discrepancies between large and small randomized trials in meta-analyses. *Ann Intern Med*, 135:11, 982–989.
6. Moher, D. et al. 1999. Improving the quality of reports of meta-analyses of randomized controlled trials: The QUORUM statement. Quality of Reporting of meta-analyses. *Lancet*, 354:9193, 1896–1899.
7. Stroup, D. F. et al. 2000. Meta-analysis of observational studies in epidemiology: A proposal for reporting. *JAMA*, 283:15, 2008–2012.
8. http://en.wikipedia.org/wiki/Clinical_trial. 2005.
9. www.clinicaltrials.gov/ct/info/phase. 2005.
10. Dr. S. Murray, lecture notes on Clinical Trials, University of Michigan School of Public Health, 2000–2001.

REVIEW QUESTIONS

1. Case–control studies start with the diagnosis and look back at associated variables, so they are done _____.

2. Case–control studies do not have a uniform starting point, so they cannot give a measure of _____ _____, but they do measure _____ _____.

3. Randomized trials do not let individuals choose their pathways, so the _____ variables should be equally distributed and not affect the outcome.

4. In a _____ trial, the subjects do not know which intervention they are getting, so they will not be biased in their response.

5. Sometimes the results of a well-executed trial are not reproducible in the _____, which may be a result of selection bias.

6. A _____ does not enroll its own subjects, but combines data that has already been collected and analyzed.

7. If a funnel diagram displays asymmetry, there may be _____ bias.

8. Once a drug is studied on human subjects, a _____ III trial is a randomized, controlled trial that compares the new drug to the standard of care.

ANSWERS TO REVIEW QUESTIONS

1. retrospectively

2. relative risk, odds ratios

3. confounding

4. blinded

5. community

6. meta-analysis

7. publication

8. phase

18

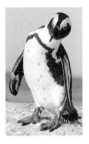

Evaluating the Evidence

Evidence-based medicine is the practice of making medical decisions through the judicious identification, evaluation, and application of the most relevant information.

—*D. J. Friedland, et al.*[1]

Medical professionals will often find themselves in the position to form an opinion or make a recommendation to a patient based on the medical literature. A courtroom judge may need to decide on the validity and admissibility of expert testimony. A journalist may need to write an article about a so-called medical breakthrough to satisfy the public's curiosity. In each case, the professional goes to the literature, hoping to find an answer. There is an overwhelming plethora of research out there. How does one begin to critique these studies?

Any well-designed study results in a solid conclusion. However, the type of study design limits the strength of the conclusion that can be drawn. A study is what it is. For example, the most precise methodology in a case–control study cannot eliminate all potential recall bias, or a meticulous cohort study could still be marred by unaccountable confounding variables. Even randomized, controlled trials have their limitations in selection and data analysis. Each type of study makes a major contribution to the fund of knowledge. The strength of the conclusion, however, is a function of the methodology and amount of bias that tags along.

The most precise study is like pure gold. Bias represents the impurities that are found in the finished product. It takes a concentrated effort to remove the impurities during the design and execution of a trial. Although some studies cannot be refined more than they are because of the inherent limitations in the design, the product can still have significant value. Bias cannot be eliminated totally but, when it is reduced as in a DBRCT, the research is more robust.

Several authors and committees have published a rating system for evaluating the strength of the evidence. For example, the U.S. Preventive Services Task Force has published a simple hierarchy of the quality of evidence based on study design (summarized in Table 18-1). In this scheme, a well-designed DBRCT described in a literature review would have more credence than an observational study. A recommendation is graded on a letter scale according to the supporting evidence in its favor. The strength of the recommendation will directly parallel the quality of evidence.

TABLE 18-1 **Rating Clinical Evidence**
Assessment System of the U.S. Preventive Services Task Force

Quality of Evidence

I	Evidence from at least one properly designed randomized, controlled trial.
II-1	Evidence obtained from well-designed controlled trials without randomization.
II-2	Evidence from well-designed cohort or case–control studies, preferably from more than one center or research group.
II-3	Evidence from multiple time series with or without the intervention. Important results in uncontrolled experiments (such as the introduction of penicillin treatment in the 1940s) could also be considered as this type of evidence.
III	Opinions of respected authorities, based on clinical experience, descriptive studies, or reports of expert committees.

Strength of Recommendations

A	Good evidence to support the intervention.
B	Fair evidence to support the intervention.
C	Insufficient evidence to recommend for or against the intervention, but recommendation might be made on other grounds.
D	Fair evidence against the intervention.
E	Good evidence against the intervention.

(From Friedland, D. J. et al. 1998. *Evidence-based medicine: a framework for clinical practice.* Stamford CT: Appleton & Lange, p. 229 with permission.)

Most published scales are in agreement with this rating system. In some of these, meta-analysis is placed at the top of the list as being the most reliable evidence.

Another approach is to rate the indication for performing a certain procedure. These guidelines ensure that the resources are appropriately distributed to those subjects who will gain the most from the intervention or test. They also attempt to identify patients who are at a higher risk of harm from the procedure. The American College of Cardiology and the American Heart Association (ACC/AHA) have implemented a classification system (summarized in Table 18-2) that is used to evaluate the indications for performing a particular procedure or treatment.

HOW TO CRITIQUE THE LITERATURE

A literature search will identify several pertinent articles. We know how to grade the evidence, but how do we go about evaluating an individual article? It helps to have

TABLE 18-2 **Classification of Recommendations**

Classifications

Class I	Conditions for which there is evidence and/or general agreement that a given procedure or treatment is useful and effective.
Class II	Conditions for which there is conflicting evidence and/or a divergence of opinion about the usefulness/efficacy of a procedure or treatment.
Class IIa	Weight of evidence/opinion is in favor of usefulness/efficacy.
Class IIb	Usefulness/efficacy is less well-established by evidence/opinion.
Class III	Conditions for which there is evidence and/or general agreement that the procedure/treatment is not useful/effective and in some cases may be harmful.

Level of Evidence

Level of Evidence A	Data derived from multiple randomized clinical trials or meta-analyses.
Level of Evidence B	Data derived from a single randomized trial or nonrandomized studies.
Level of Evidence C	Only consensus opinion of experts, case studies, or standard-of-care.

(Adapted from www.acc.org/qualityandscience/clinical/statements, 2006.)

an organized approach when critiquing the literature. At this point, you now have the skills to do this with confidence. Various methods to evaluate a study have been proposed; some experts recommend a specific approach based on the study design. This results in an in-depth critique of the study and is useful for intensive reviews of the literature, such as during "journal club" meetings. However, these approaches require a significant time commitment and continuous reference to a printed set of guidelines. It may not be necessary to critique every article with such scrutiny. I would like to propose a simple method that is applicable to any type of study. It does not require a printed checklist or template.

W W H W W

Notice that this is a palindrome—a symmetrical display of letters that reads the same forward or backward. This is a memory trick. These represent five questions you should ask yourself whenever you evaluate a study:

WHY was the study done? This can often be found in the title of the article. It reflects the research hypothesis. The introduction educates the reader about the existing information in the field and justifies the efforts of the investigators and subjects. The research hypothesis is often a very specific question that serves to fill in a piece of a larger puzzle.

WHO was being studied? This is found in the inclusion and exclusion criteria. It is the definition of the population. It identifies the type of individual who may benefit from the knowledge.

HOW was the study done? This is the nuts and bolts of the article. The specifics can be found in the Methods section. How were the subjects recruited? How was the study set up to answer the research hypothesis? Ask yourself whether it is an observational study or a controlled trial, keeping in mind the limitations of each type of design. If it was a prospective trial, for how long were the subjects followed?

WHAT were the results? This is found in the Results section of the article. The outcome measure (such as relative risk or odds ratio) with a *p* value should be mentioned, as well as results for analyses done on subgroups. A wider confidence interval for the outcomes measure will reflect a larger margin of error for estimating the true value of the population parameter.

WHERE were the potential sources of bias? These are the limitations of the study. Most authors will address these issues in the Discussion section, but you might identify a few concerns of your own. Remember, bias cannot be totally eliminated from any study but certain trial designs can minimize it. It also behooves the reader to see who funded the study. A potential source of bias exists when the financing is provided by an individual or a corporation that would stand to benefit from the result.

EVIDENCE-BASED MEDICINE AND YOU

We have now reached the point where we have learned the skills we need to navigate through the medical literature. We know how and why samples are used to study populations. We know the theory behind the statistical tests used to test the null hypothesis, and how we use sampling distributions to calculate the probability of the observed result. We are comfortable in the definition of a *p* value (remember, you are a PRO) and with the umbrella concept of the confidence interval. We also explored some philosophical issues and looked at the history of the development of medical research. The reason we went through the trouble of learning these things, of course, is so we can all contribute to decisions that allow people to live longer and feel better.

Dave Sackett is a physician in the United Kingdom who has long been a champion for the cause of applying evidence-based medicine to our professional practices. The fact that he is placed at the end of this section in no way underestimates the significant contributions he has made in this arena. He has devoted his professional career to promoting the process of medical decision-making based on the best evidence. He outlines the five steps[2] we must take to incorporate this approach into the way we perform our jobs:

1. Convert information needs into answerable questions.
2. Track down the best evidence with which to answer them.
3. Critically appraise that evidence for its validity and usefulness.
4. Apply the results in our practice.
5. Evaluate our performance.

These statements pretty much sum up the objectives of this book, one of which is to provide you with the skill necessary to interpret the medical literature. This will give you the confidence you need to practice evidence-based medicine. Now that you understand the approach, you may feel a paradigm shift taking place when you encounter medical problems. You will find that the literature is your best friend when you need to make a decision. This reliable resource is readily available and hopefully not nearly as intimidating now as it used to be. Enjoy using your new knowledge.

May you live long and feel good!

KEY POINTS

- One commonly accepted scale in rating the quality of the literature is based on the design of the study.
- The quality of the available evidence is used to rate the strength of a recommendation. These recommendations take into account who will benefit the most from a given intervention, who will benefit the least, and who is likely to be harmed.
- An easy approach to evaluating an individual article is W W H W W:
  - Why is the study being done?
  - Who is the population?
  - How was the study done?
  - What were the results?
  - Where are the potential sources of bias?
- Evidence-based medicine uses the skills you have just learned to integrate validated knowledge into medical practice so people may live longer and feel better, and so resources may be distributed fairly.

REFERENCES

1. Friedland, D. J. et al. 1998. *Evidence-based medicine: a framework for clinical practice.* Stamford CT: Appleton & Lange.
2. Sackett D. L. et al. 1996. *Evidence-based medicine: how to practice and teach EPBM.* New York, NY: Churchill Livingstone.

REVIEW QUESTION

1. Now that I can evaluate the literature, I feel comfortable using it to make decisions that help people _____ _____ and _____ _____.

ANSWER TO REVIEW QUESTION

1. live longer, feel better

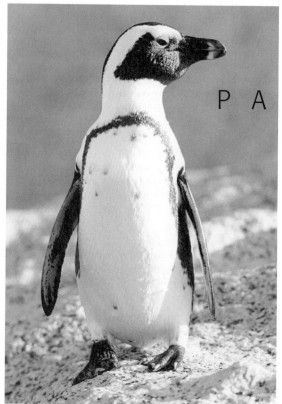

Common Applications

Statistics is both an art and a science.
—*M. Anthony Schork and Richard D. Remington*[1]

INTRODUCTION TO PART III

The first step in a research study is to ask a pertinent question. The outcome measure that is chosen depends on the type of study that is being constructed. There are many applications of data that can result in a variety of outcome measures to estimate population parameters for the final analysis. There may be more than one correct approach.

The next chapter describes the more familiar measures and how they are used to compare results, especially when trying to estimate a parameter such as risk. The basic concept of economic analysis is also presented. This is an emerging statistical technique which quantifies cost along with benefit. The last chapter focuses on the different ways to assess the accuracy of medical tests that are performed on patients that have an impact on the treatment decisions.

These chapters are meant to be used as a reference. When you come across a particular type of study or diagnostic test, read the synopsis on the subject to understand how to interpret the results and familiarize yourself with its applications. If you want to learn more about a particular subject, you will need to consult a formal Statistics or Epidemiology textbook.

REFERENCE

1. Schork, M. A. and Remington, R. D. 2000. *Statistics with applications to the biological and health sciences*, 3rd ed. Upper Saddle River, NJ: Prentice Hall, p 5.

CHAPTER **19**

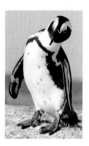

Measures of Effect

Making decisions is the most important part of most jobs.

—*Robert Hooke*[1]

When we estimate a parameter, we are often attempting to estimate the strength of a relationship or the magnitude of an effect of one variable upon another. Even if we have determined that the data support a significant effect, it is helpful to estimate the extent of that effect. For example, in a study comparing a Standard of Care Drug with a New Drug, both interventions may have a positive result but we would like to know the degree of benefit of one pathway over the other. The measures that are used depend on the design of the study.

ODDS RATIO

This type of measure is used in case–control studies. In the metaphor of the train station, case–control studies start out at the Disease destinations such as Cancer and No Cancer. We then look back to see what the individuals in these groups had packed in their suitcases (or what they were exposed to). We compare the number of individuals in each group who have packed a certain item, such as cigarettes.

The odds of having an exposure is the probability of having had an exposure divided by the probability of not having had the exposure. For example, in patients with a certain type of lung cancer, the odds of having been exposed to cigarettes are:

$$\text{Odds} = \frac{\text{Probability of exposure to cigarettes}}{\text{Probability of no exposure to cigarettes}}$$

The same calculation can be done for subjects who are healthy. Both groups have some degree of exposure. When we compare the fractions, as shown in Figure 19-1, we are comparing the odds that cancer subjects were exposed to cigarettes versus the odds that the healthy controls were exposed. This is known as the *odds ratio*.

If there is no difference in exposure, the result will be close to 1, which supports the conclusion that the exposure has no association with the disease. The farther the odds ratio is from 1, the stronger the association. Using the formula in Figure 19-1,

	Cases (With Disease)	Controls (Without Disease)
History of Exposure	a	b
No History of Exposure	c	d

FIGURE 19-1 In an odds ratio, we first divide the groups into diseased versus normal, as indicated by the double line. Then we look at the numbers who were exposed in each group versus nonexposed. The end result gives us the odds that cases were exposed compared to the odds that controls were exposed. (Adapted from Gordis, L. 2001. Epidemiology, 3rd ed., Philadelphia: Elsevier.)

$$\text{Odds Ratio} = \frac{\text{Odds that a case was exposed}}{\text{Odds that a control was exposed}}$$

$$= \frac{a/c}{b/d} = \frac{ad}{bc}$$

a number greater than 1 supports an association between cigarette exposure and lung cancer. In some cases, the exposure may be protective, such as the exposure of seat belt use in subjects who suffered car crash mortalities versus those who lived. In this case, the odds ratio would be smaller than 1, which would indicate that the odds of having used a seat belt in car crash mortality victims are less than the odds of seat belt use in those who survived a car crash.

The odds ratio is not a measure of risk. Recall that risk is the rate of occurrence of an event over time. Case–control studies cannot provide this information; since they are retrospective studies, there is no true starting point in time. However, the odds ratio in a retrospective study will approximate the risk of disease if the incidence of the disease is fairly low in the population.

It is also possible to use a prospective study to calculate an odds ratio. This scenario is shown in Figure 19-2. The relative odds in both case–control and cohort studies results in the same number. It is an effective way to measure whether a specific exposure is associated with a disease.

The odds ratio is often reported as a single number followed by a confidence interval in parentheses. On a graph, the confidence interval may be represented by a bar. If the range of the confidence interval includes the number 1, then the result was not found to be statistically significant. Figure 19-3 is an illustration of the odds ratios from a few studies that looked at short-term mortality in patients with acute myocardial infarction (AMI) and the benefit of starting a medication called an angiotensin-converting enzyme (ACE) inhibitor in these individuals.

RELATIVE RISK

The measurement of risk captures the probability that a particular event or outcome will happen over time. Thus, risk can only be determined from a study that looks at subjects prospectively. Risk ratios compare the risk for two or more groups.

	Develop Disease	Do Not Develop Disease
Exposed	a	b
Not Exposed	c	d

$$\text{Odds Ratio} = \frac{\text{Odds that an exposed person develops disease}}{\text{Odds that a nonexposed person develops disease}}$$

$$= \frac{a/b}{c/d} = \frac{ad}{bc}$$

FIGURE 19-2 The odds ratio can be derived from a cohort study. The formula is ultimately the same as the odds ratio in a case–control study, but we compare the odds of developing disease in the exposed group versus the nonexposed controls. *(Adapted from Gordis, L. 2001. Epidemiology, 3rd ed., Philadelphia: Elsevier.)*

$$\text{Relative risk} = \frac{\text{Incidence of disease in exposed}}{\text{Incidence of disease in nonexposed}}$$

When we calculate a risk ratio, we are comparing the incidence of disease in the exposed group to the incidence of disease in the nonexposed group. The familiar 2×2 table in Figure 19-4 illustrates how the calculation is done.

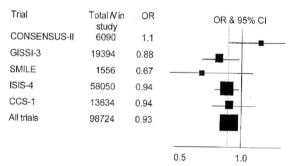

Trial	Total N in study	OR	OR & 95% CI
CONSENSUS-II	6090	1.1	
GISSI-3	19394	0.88	
SMILE	1556	0.67	
ISIS-4	58050	0.94	
CCS-1	13634	0.94	
All trials	98724	0.93	

0.5   1.0

FIGURE 19-3 The odds ratios of being exposed to an ACE inhibitor in those with short-term survival after an AMI versus those who died. The CONSENSUS-II study used an intravenous preparation, whereas an oral preparation was used in the other studies. The size of the box is proportional to the number of subjects. If a confidence interval line crosses 1, the results are not significant. We know that if a study is underpowered we may not pick up a significant effect even if one exists (a Type II error). When the data are combined, the true odds ratio can be more accurately estimated. These results suggest a true survival benefit from the early administration of an ACE inhibitor in AMI. *(Data from Zipes, D. P. et al. 2004. Braunwald's Heart Disease, 7th ed. Philadelphia: Elsevier/Saunders, p. 1192.)*

	Develop Disease	Do Not Develop Disease
Exposed	a	b
Not Exposed	c	d

Incidence Rates of Disease

in exposed: $\frac{a}{a+b}$

in nonexposed: $\frac{c}{c+d}$

$$\text{Risk ratio} = \frac{\frac{a}{a+b}}{\frac{c}{c+d}}$$

FIGURE 19-4 The risk ratio, or relative risk, compares the incidence of disease in the exposed versus the nonexposed individuals. *(Adapted from Gordis, L. 2001.* Epidemiology, *3rd ed., Philadelphia: Elsevier.)*

The interpretation of relative risk is similar to that of the odds ratio. If the relative risk is close to 1, there is no association between exposure and development of disease. A relative risk greater than 1 indicates a positive association between the exposure and the disease. A relative risk less than 1 means the exposure is associated with less disease, and may be protective. Figure 19-5 shows the effect of a class of drug known as beta blockers in the treatment of AMI. The relative risk of mortality is compared in those who were given this drug versus those who were not.

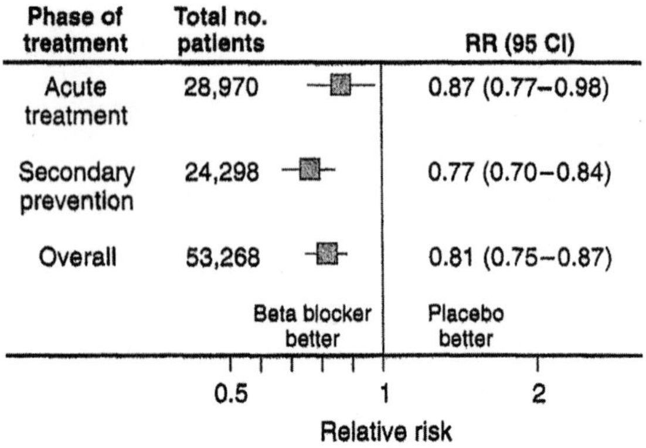

FIGURE 19-5 Effect of beta blockers on mortality rate in patients with myocardial infarction. The relative risk of mortality is reduced with beta blockers both during the acute phase of treatment and when prescribed as secondary prevention after AMI. *(Data from Zipes, D. P. et al. 2004.* Braunwald's Heart Disease, *7th ed. Philadelphia: Elsevier/Saunders, p. 1190.)*

ABSOLUTE RISK AND ATTRIBUTABLE RISK

Relative risk considers the fact that some disease occurs in nonexposed individuals, such as the incidence of lung cancer in non-smokers. It reflects the increased amount of disease seen in the exposed individuals (or decreased amount of disease when the exposure is protective). The relative risk is a measure of the strength of the association.

The background risk in nonexposed individuals is known as the *absolute risk*. Another useful measure is the additional amount of disease in the population that is seen due to the exposure of certain individuals, called the *attributable risk*. This measure takes into account the disease burden on the community and how much disease can be prevented if the exposure is eliminated. The incidence of disease that is attributed to an exposure is calculated as:

$$\text{Attributable risk} = \frac{(\text{Incidence in exposed group})}{(\text{Incidence in nonexposed group})}$$

If there is a strong association between exposure and the development of disease, the attributable risk will be high. Removing the exposure will have a significant impact on the overall incidence of the disease and the burden on the health care system. One can also express the attributable risk as the proportion of additional risk in exposed individuals, which can be expressed as a percentage. The formula for this is:

$$\frac{(\text{Incidence in exposed group}) - (\text{incidence in non-exposed group})}{\text{Incidence in exposed group}}$$

RISK REDUCTION

Some exposures are protective and result in better outcomes, as we saw in the data on beta blocker and ACE inhibitor medications for patients with AMI. The absolute risk reduction looks at the decrease in the overall incidence of disease or death for those receiving the therapy. The formula is:

$$\text{Absolute risk reduction} = (\text{Incidence in placebo group}) - (\text{incidence in treatment group})$$

The relative risk reduction for a therapy can seem quite large but, when it is applied to the population and the absolute risk reduction is calculated, the benefit may be modest at best. This happens when the therapy works well but the incidence of disease in the placebo group is small to begin with. Consider the following example of a new medication that is being tested for its ability to prevent renal toxicity in subjects who are given a contrast agent (such as iodine) during a computed tomography (CT) scan. The study looks at 200 people undergoing a contrast CT scan. Half get the new medicine and half get placebo, and the incidence of renal toxicity is observed.

$$N = 200$$

	Toxicity	No Toxicity
New Medicine	2	98
Placebo	4	96

Relative Risk
Reduction: $\dfrac{\text{Medication } \dfrac{2}{100}}{\text{Placebo } \dfrac{4}{100}} = \dfrac{.02}{.04} = .5 \text{ or } 50\%$

Absolute Risk
Reduction: $\dfrac{\text{Placebo}}{\dfrac{4}{100}} - \dfrac{\text{Medication}}{\dfrac{2}{100}} = \dfrac{2}{100} = 0.02 \text{ or } 2\%$

The incidence of renal toxicity is 4/100 in the placebo group, and 2/100 in the treatment group. The medication reduced the number of events by half, so the relative risk reduction is 50%, which seems like quite a lot. The absolute risk reduction considers the rate of events in the population. Taken in this context, the medication reduced events by 2%, which is a more reasonable measure of performance in a population.

NUMBER NEEDED TO TREAT

The reduction in absolute risk takes into account the number of events that occur in a population with and without treatment. This means that events will happen whether or not we intervene, but we can reduce this rate with an effective treatment. It also means that some people will get the treatment who would not have had an event anyway. A more intuitive way to express this number is by *number needed to treat* (NNT). It reflects the number of people who will get the treatment who would not have had an event, for every one person in which the event is prevented. The NNT is the reciprocal of the absolute risk reduction. The formula is:

$$\text{NNT} = \frac{1}{(\text{Incidence in placebo group}) - (\text{incidence in treatment group})}$$

NNT gives us an idea of how many people will need to be exposed to the treatment so that we may reap the benefit in one individual. In the above example regarding the prevention of renal toxicity in contrast CT scans, the NNT = 1/0.02 or 50. We would need to treat 50 people to prevent one event.

Even though NNT does not take into account the cost or side effects of the treatment, we make a mental note of these when using this measure. If the treatment is safe and cheap, we are more likely to recommend it even if the NNT is relatively large. Keep in mind that we can reduce the NNT when we tailor the population we treat. For instance, we know that diabetics and people with pre-existing kidney disease have a higher incidence of renal toxicity to contrast agents. If we restricted the use of the preventive medication to these individuals, we are likely to see a larger absolute risk reduction and therefore a smaller NNT.

KAPLAN–MEIER SURVIVAL CURVES

If we follow two groups of subjects over a demarcated period of time, we can analyze the survival benefit by comparing the proportions of those who are alive in each group at the end of the time period. However, many studies that track mortality enroll patients at several different entry times and follow them for different lengths of time. The Kaplan–Meier method of survival analysis is frequently used for analyzing these types of longitudinal studies. In contrast to methods that calculate survival rates over fixed time intervals, such as actuarial tables, this measure calculates a new survival rate every time a death occurs. Because the deaths do not occur consistently, there are irregular time intervals; the graph looks like uneven steps. The graph plots the proportion of surviving subjects every time a death occurs, and is essentially the probability of survival at any given time interval starting from time zero (when the subject entered the study).

These studies are often done over many years, so it is not unusual to lose track of some of the subjects. The length of time that they were observed, however, provides important information. The Kaplan–Meier analysis accounts for those lost to follow-up (referred to as *censored* data) by assigning the weighted probability of death in these subjects based on the death rates in those who remained under observation. It incorporates these data when the probability of survival is recalculated each time a death occurs.

When two or more groups are being studied, the curves are plotted together. The slopes of the curves can be compared using a statistical analysis such as the log rank test. If the curves are close, or cross, they are unlikely to have significantly different survival rates and the two pathways being studied will have equal benefit. Figure 19-6 is an example of a Kaplan–Meier curve in women with breast cancer who were randomized to participate in either the supportive-expressive group therapy or the control group. Even though the curves are different, there was no significant difference in survival in the two groups ($p = 0.72$).

On occasion you will see event-free survival plotted on the ordinate. If someone is alive but has an event that is being monitored, such as a stroke, this will result in a drop in the curve. Besides tracking survival versus no survival, this method is also used for other dichotomous outcomes that occur over time, such as the development of diabetes versus no diabetes.

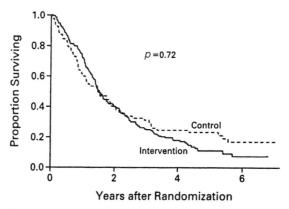

FIGURE 19-6 Kaplan–Meier survival curves for women assigned to the intervention group and the control group. There was no significant difference in survival between the two groups. *(Adapted from Gordis, L. 2001. Epidemiology, 3rd ed., Philadelphia: Elsevier.)*

COX PROPORTIONAL HAZARDS ANALYSIS

This methodology is used to test for differences in survival, but at the same time accounts for other variables that might affect the outcome but could not be controlled when the subjects were enrolled. For instance, age of the subjects at the time of entry into a study could influence the difference in survival rates if one group enrolled significantly older individuals than the other. The Cox method allows us to identify which variables are associated with better survival. It can also be used to quantify the effect of multiple variables on other dichotomous outcomes, such as body weight and dietary habits in the development of diabetes versus no diabetes.

The *hazard ratio* is a comparison of the effect of different variables on survival or other outcomes that develop over time. It is similar to a risk ratio in that the higher the hazard ratio, the greater the probability that the exposed individual will develop the outcome compared to those without the exposure.

REFERENCE

1. Hooke, R. 1983. *How to tell the liars from the statisticians.* New York: Marcel Dekker, Inc.

CHAPTER **20**

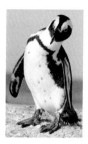

Economic Analysis

Resources used to provide health care are vast, but not limitless.

—*Mike F. Drummond et al.*[1]

The measures of effect we have considered so far are purely scientific. They steer us toward a particular pathway on the noble principle of providing live longer/feel better outcomes to improve people's existence. Yet we live in a world of limited resources, so practicing medicine effectively requires some degree of economic consideration. As the population increases and ages, the cost of treatment will continue to rise, especially for conditions that are prevalent and relatively expensive to treat. Economic analysis is an approach that takes into account not only the live longer/feel better measure but also the cost of implementing various interventions.

Cost-effectiveness is a type of economic analysis that quantifies benefit through one of the standard outcome measures that capture mortality, or quality of life (QOL). The measure can reflect reduced QOL that might result from medication side effects, worsening disease, or from a complication of a procedure that would affect overall well-being. In addition, the financial cost of going down this pathway is taken into consideration. This includes not only the up-front costs of a procedure and medication, but can also account for hidden costs from a societal perspective, such as lost income due to inability to work or the cost of a caretaker while a patient is recuperating. *Cost-utility* studies specifically account for the number of years lived in full health (QUALY), and are considered a type of cost-effective analysis, but the two are often used interchangeably.[2]

For instance, let us consider a theoretical situation of an expensive surgical procedure that improves eyesight in a prevalent condition that causes impaired vision. The patients can also use eyedrops and get improvement, but their vision improves more if they have the operation. So far, it seems like the operation should be recommended. However, what if several procedures over a number of months were needed to produce the desired result, and each operation carried a small but definite risk of permanent blindness in that eye? What would be the comparative cost and benefit of each pathway? Now the decision is not so straightforward. Let us try to approach this problem using economic analysis.

First, it is important to know that many of these studies look at cost and benefit over several years, often until the subjects have all died from either a complication of their illness or some other cause. Since the exact data are often not available, these models incorporate the available data based on observations of subjects (over several years) who have gone down the various pathways. Simulations are then done on computer programs that project these data into the future, for the rest of the subjects' lives.

The compared outcomes include cost and benefit for each pathway. The formula for comparison is:

$$\frac{\text{Cost of pathway 2} - \text{cost of pathway 1}}{\text{Outcome of pathway 2} - \text{outcome of pathway 1}}$$

The outcome data are taken from published trials or other databases (or expert opinion when the above are not available). If we wanted to consider mortality in the above example, we would go to the literature to find the mortality rate for the eye surgery. Otherwise, if the disease has no effect on mortality, we assume that person will live to the expected average age for their gender and disease state. These data can often be found in actuarial tables provided by life insurance companies.

Our outcome measure should also capture QOL. Since QOL is strongly linked to vision, we can use an objective measure such as a vision test to quantify this. In addition, we can consider the impact on QOL for blindness in that eye if a subject undergoes the surgery and suffers this complication. If the surgery is done more than once, the potential impact of this complication should be taken into consideration each time.

A relative point system is used to quantify QOL. Again, these data are usually taken from published surveys found in the literature. In the above example, QOL for one year after losing the sight in one eye may be 0.7 on a relative scale of 0 to 1, with 0 = death and 1 = full health. For someone who avoids surgery and uses eyedrops, the continued impairment in their vision might give them a QOL = 0.5. If their vision deteriorated to a point where they were unable to drive or earn an income, the QOL would be even lower.

Because QOL is subjective, the assigned value for a given disease state (such as blindness) may vary from one person to another. For instance, it is quite possible that someone who loses their eyesight may report a worse QOL than someone who was born blind. Accurate measurements of QOL depend on many observations from large populations.

Measuring costs can be challenging for several reasons. The cost of providing a service or product is not necessarily what the consumer is charged. In addition, what is billed is not always collected. Medical costs that are accrued in a hospital are fairly straightforward; they are tabulated from what is reimbursed to the hospital and physicians through insurance companies. However, this does require a thorough understanding of the complex billing and reimbursement process. The costs of outpatient visits, medical equipment, pharmaceuticals, and transportation to and from appointments are also considered. If there is a probability of needing nursing home care, this should be accounted for. Lost wages because of illness also need to be assessed. When projections are made into the future, the figures need to be adjusted for inflation. Prevalent conditions or costly interventions are more likely to be studied because their cost to society is so much greater compared to other conditions having less financial impact.

How do we incorporate all these figures into the above formula? We start with a decision tree, which compares the pathways. This is a graph that accounts for all possible outcomes. A circle (node) is used to represent an intervention that could have more than one outcome. When an intervention is done, the subjects are divided at the node and the number of subjects who continue down a particular path will depend on the chance of the event occurring.

Figure 20-1 is a simplified decision tree from the example on impaired vision. All the subjects are from the same population and meet the inclusion and exclusion criteria.

Theoretically, if 100 patients went down each pathway we could tabulate costs and quantify the benefit for each arm. We need to know the probability of improved vision, same vision, and decreased vision for each intervention. (This example assumes that the mortality from the surgery is negligible.) We also need to know the probability of blindness as a complication of surgery. Those who underwent surgery and had no change in their vision or had worsening vision will undergo a second operation, so they will funnel back through the node. We can elect to stop the process at any given point in time. If we want to follow the subjects for 10 years, we can project the data to that point. It is also possible to simulate the process until everyone has died.

The benefit includes the QOL measures we considered earlier. The benefit will be greater in the surgical arm because more people have improved vision. However, the benefit to those using eyedrops is not insignificant, since 25% will improve with the drops alone.

We mentioned that the surgery is expensive and some subjects have it multiple times. The cost in the surgical arm will thus be high. It is also possible that the cost in the eyedrops arm will be high if the drops are expensive and need to be dosed several times a day, or if a substantial number of subjects ultimately need continuous assistance because of deteriorating vision. It is difficult to predict which arm will have a more favorable cost/benefit ratio, but that is exactly the sort of question that economic analysis attempts to answer.

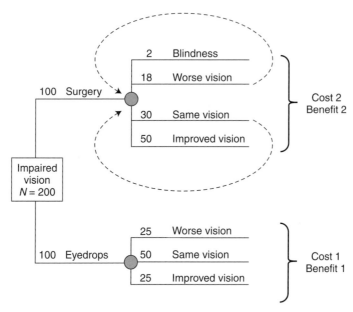

FIGURE 20-1 Decision tree for eye surgery versus medical treatment.

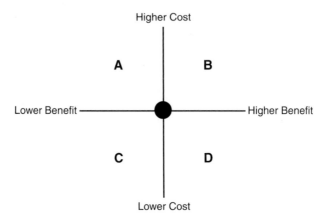

FIGURE 20-2 The advantage of an alternate pathway relative to the current standard of care pathway when considering cost and benefit. A number that falls into quadrant A reflects lower benefit at a higher cost, and therefore this pathway should be abandoned. A result that falls into quadrant D is a no-brainer—the alternate pathway is better *and* cheaper, and should be recommended. The recommendations for results in quadrants B and C are less clear and require discussion as to whether the cost of the alternate treatment justifies the benefit (quadrant B) or whether cost containment is worth the incremental loss of benefit (quadrant C). *(From class notes on Economic Analysis, Prof. Michael Chernow, University of Michigan School of Public Health, 2000.)*

The costs and benefits are summed for each pathway through a complex formula that also weight the result by the probability of each event occurring. The final result is a quantitative representation of the cost of a pathway for a unit of benefit, such as one quality-adjusted life-year (QUALY). It is intuitive that a pathway with a better result will often cost more. In this situation, it is up to society to decide whether the cost justifies the benefit. Figure 20-2 is a graph that plots incremental cost to benefit of an alternate pathway compared to the standard of care, which is assigned a baseline cost/benefit in the middle of the graph.

The strength of economic analysis is limited by the availability of data. The process requires integration of the results of several trials. The data used in the comparisons of various pathways might be from trials in which the populations were not exactly the same or different treatment paths were considered. The cost estimates can differ based on the source of information and perspective (e.g., using cost figures based on what is charged versus what is collected). Inherent in this type of study is the fact that a number of assumptions will be made. One way to approach the uncertainty of the projected cost and benefit is to do a *sensitivity analysis*. This employs a range of values for certain key variables. For instance, if the complication rate for a procedure can be kept very low (hence improving QOL and decreasing the cost for one pathway), the intervention may cross the threshold point at which it is considered cost-effective. The sensitivity analysis looks at several values for the variables that could have an impact on the results and ultimate recommendations.

REFERENCE

1. Drummond, M. F. et al. 1997. Users' Guide to the Medical Literature, *JAMA*, 277:10.
2. wikipedia.org/wiki/cost-utility_analysis 2007.

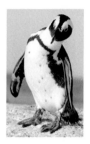

CHAPTER 21

Assessment of Tests

Diagnostic tests are most useful when they change a probability across a decision-making threshold.

Lee Goldman et al.[1]

We use measures of accuracy to determine the reliability of a test result. This information comes from studying a sample from a population of individuals defined by inclusion and exclusion criteria. For instance, people often present to the health care system with symptoms of chest pain. If we excluded those younger than age 18 and studied a sample of these folks by giving each of them two tests—the definitive Reference Standard and the test under consideration—we would know how accurate the test is by comparing it to the results of the Reference Standard.

Either the individual has the Disease (D) or is Normal (N). Only the Reference Standard can precisely tell us that. This test is the most reliable in distinguishing D from N, but is often invasive and expensive. Because of this, it is not the first test to perform. When we see patients, we do not know whether they are D or N. Sometimes we can rely solely on symptoms and signs to arrive at a diagnosis; for example, a patient with symptoms and signs of uncomplicated gastritis can often be treated medically without exposure to further testing. In other cases, however, we want to be more assured of the diagnosis, especially if the treatment is expensive, extended, or has significant side effects.

The tests we use will either be positive (+) or negative (−). Not all subjects who test + will have D, and not all those who test − will be Normal. There will be false positives and false negatives, but an accurate test will have minimal false results. The following 2 × 2 table shows how subjects with D and N could be distributed among those being tested.

	Disease State	
	Disease	Normal
+	True positive	False positive
−	False negative	True negative

Test Result

SENSITIVITY AND SPECIFICITY

Sensitivity is the probability that someone with D will test positive. It is the number of true positives divided by all those with D, which includes not only those who are D and test positive (the true positives) but also those who are D and test negative (the false negatives). Notice that sensitivity is only concerned with those in the D column of the above table.

The formula for sensitivity is:

$$\text{Sensitivity} = \frac{\text{True Positives}}{\text{True Positives} + \text{False Negatives}}$$

Specificity, on the other hand, is the probability that someone who is N will test negative. It is the number of true negatives divided by all those who are N, which includes both true negatives and false positives. Specificity is concerned with only those in the N column.

The formula for specificity is:

$$\text{Specificity} = \frac{\text{True Negatives}}{\text{True Negatives} + \text{False Positives}}$$

One way to understand sensitivity and specificity is to split the columns, as in the following table, because those with the disease do not overlap with the normal individuals.

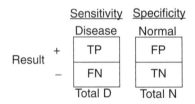

The concepts of sensitivity and specificity are counterintuitive because patients do not present with a sign that identifies them as either D or N, but they can undergo testing that places them in either the positive or negative row. As we will see, positive and negative predictive values may be more useful when deciding whether or not a patient has a disease based on the test results.

It is interesting that these tests rule disease in or out through a circuitous process. A highly sensitive test will approach 100% sensitivity. This means the value of the numerator will be very close to that of the denominator. This, in turn, means the number of false negatives will be very low. Compared to all the negative results, then, a negative test will be believable. A negative result will reliably indicate someone who is N. For a test with a high sensitivity, a negative result rules the disease out.

SnNOut: high Sensitivity, Negative test rules it Out.[2]

On the other hand, a highly specific test will not have many false positives, and those who do test positive are likely to be true positives, or Ds. For a highly specific test with a positive result, the individual is likely to have the disease.

SpPIn: high <u>Sp</u>ecificity, <u>P</u>ositive test rules it <u>In</u>.[2]

If you remember SnNOut and SpPIn, you will be able to apply these tests in the appropriate settings. When considering the sensitivity and specificity of a test, always ask yourself "What is the Reference Standard that the test was compared to?" (keeping in mind that some Reference Standard tests may not be 100% accurate). Also note the population that was studied when the sensitivity and specificity of the test were being determined. Individuals were found to be either N or D by the Reference Standard, but they all had to meet the same inclusion and exclusion criteria to be considered in the comparison. Certain populations with risk factors for the disease will have an increased proportion of D, which can result in an exaggerated ability of the test to pick up those cases.

BOX 21-1

The Shepherd Story

Sensitivity and specificity are easier to understand if we use a metaphor. Think of two types of shepherds, each caring over a flock of Domestic animals (D) such as sheep. Each wants to build a fence around his flock to ensure that they are fed. The problem is that there are some Native animals (N), such as mice, rabbits, foxes, raccoons, etc., that are mixed in with the sheep (D). For this metaphor, consider anything inside the fence to be a + result. Anything outside the fence is a – result. The true positives will be sheep (Ds) inside the fence and true negatives will be native animals (Ns) outside the fence. A false positive will be an N inside the fence and a false negative will be represented by a D outside the fence.

A highly SENSITIVE shepherd is gENerous. He wants to be sure each of his flock D is well fed. He knows that he can build an enclosure to include each D, but he will include a few Ns as well since these are mixed in with the Ds. He also knows that anything outside the fence will definitely be an N. Connect the dashed lines to draw a fence around this flock, including all the Ds and excluding some of the Ns.

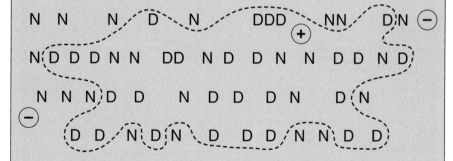

Focus on the outside of the fence, which is analogous to a negative result. A false negative would be a sheep (D) that is outside the fence. Notice, however, that outside the fence all are Ns (there are no Ds), so there are no false negatives.

- *In a highly seNsitive test, those who test Negative are likely to be truly Negative (Normal).*

Continued

BOX 21-1—cont'd

Now take the opposite approach. A highly SPECIFIC shepherd is PICky. He does not want to feed any extra animals. He builds a much more constrained fence, so that only Ds are included inside. The trade-off is that some Ds will be on the outside but anything on the inside (+) will be D. Connect the dashed lines to include only Ds inside the fence.

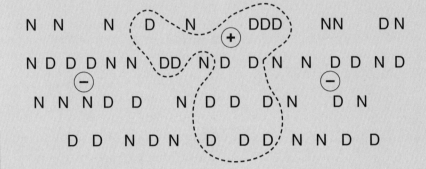

The inside of the fence is analogous to a positive result. Notice that only Ds are inside the fence so there are no false positives, although there are many false negatives which are the Ds on the outside.

- *In a highly sPecific test, those who test Positive are likely to be truly Positive (Disease).*

SCREENING TESTS

Tests can be used for diagnostic purposes in symptomatic individuals, but can also be used for screening a healthy population. Screening tests should be relatively safe, inexpensive, and simple to use. Considering the shepherd metaphor, if you wanted to screen for a disease D, which would be the most preferable test to use: one with high sensitivity or high specificity? (Clue: screening tests should be all-inclusive and not miss anyone with possible D.)

We read the test as either positive (inside the fence) or negative (outside the fence). When screening for D, we do not want to miss anyone with D so we want all the Ds to test positive, which may include a few false positives as well. We want a highly sensitive test as an initial screening tool since it will identify the true positives among all the positive results. To confirm the true presence of Ds, we can use a more specific test on those individuals whose initial screening test was positive.

RECEIVER OPERATING CHARACTERISTIC CURVES

It is very common for a test to have a range of values for the result. Whether the test is considered positive or negative depends on where we draw the line for a normal result (or how constraining our fence is). Thyroid levels, cholesterol levels, and blood pressure measurements are all examples of these tests. Figure 21-1 shows the distributions of results that we could obtain for people who are D or N.

We want a cutoff point that minimizes both the false negatives and false positives. Ideally, we would like 100% sensitivity and specificity, but we often have to settle for less than that. An increase in sensitivity is often at the expense of a decrease in specificity. A Receiver Operating Characteristic (ROC) curve can help choose the best cutoff point by graphically showing the trade-off between sensitivity and specificity.

ROC curves plot the true positive rate against the false positive rate for tests that result in a range of values, to determine the most accurate cutoff point. The name comes from a system used by the British during World War II to distinguish true radio signals from background noise. They used these graphs to evaluate their ability to accurately read signals that alerted them to a German air invasion. If they were correct, this was a true positive; if incorrect, it was a false positive. The goal of their defense system was to minimize false readings. ROC curves have also been used to evaluate the accuracy of Internet search engines.[3,4]

Figure 21-2 illustrates some ROC curves. In the evaluation of diagnostic tests, {sensitivity} is plotted on the ordinate against {1 − specificity} on the abscissa. The highest sensitivity is 100%, denoted as 1, and the highest specificity of 1 results in {1 − specificity} = 0. The most accurate tests will have a point that approaches the upper left-hand part of the graph where {sensitivity} = 1 and {1 − specificity} = 0. The least accurate tests will perform no better than chance results, represented by a straight line at a 45-degree slope.

The graph is created by plotting {1 − specificity} against {sensitivity} for different cutoff points. The closer the curve gets to the upper left-hand side of the graph, the more accurate the test is for that cutoff point. In Figure 21-2, ROC curve A illustrates a test with a near perfect sensitivity and specificity, along with other ROC curves that are more likely to be encountered.

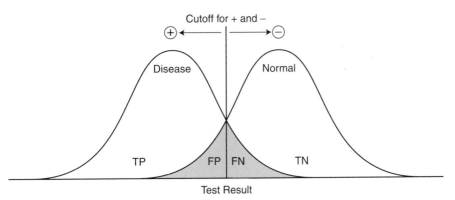

FIGURE 21-1 The distribution of test results on a continuous scale for those who are D and N. The values overlap; the distinction between a positive and negative test depends on where we draw the cutoff point. As we move it in either direction, the number of false negatives and false positives will change, which affects sensitivity and specificity. TP, true positive; FP, false positive; FN, false negative; TN, true negative. (*From www.wikipedia.org/image:Roc-general 2008.*)

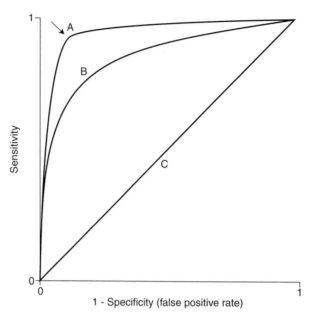

FIGURE 21-2 A, The ROC curve of a test that approaches 100% sensitivity and specificity for a cutoff point by the arrow. This is an ideal situation that is not very often encountered, and approaches the accuracy of the Reference Standard; B, A test with highest sensitivity and specificity at the point where the curve is closest to the upper left corner. This is the cutoff value that minimizes the false positives and negatives; C, A test with results no better than chance. A positive or negative slope of this line does *not at all* distinguish between D and N. (*From uptodate.com/ROC curve 2008.*)

One way to measure the accuracy of different tests, which considers both sensitivity and specificity, is to compare the areas under the curves. The total area of the graph is = 1, so a perfect test will have an area = 1. The closer the area for a particular test is to 1, the better the test. For a test with results that are no better than chance (as in curve C in Figure 21-2), the area will be 0.5.[5]

PREDICTIVE VALUES AND LIKELIHOOD RATIOS

When patients present to the health care system, they have a collection of symptoms that suggest a particular illness. Diagnostic tests help us to decide whether or not they have the disease. Tests can be compared to the Reference Standard to determine their accuracy. A *positive predictive value* is the probability that a patient who tests positive for the disease actually has it. A *negative predictive value* is the probability that someone who tests negative is truly normal. These are analogous to sensitivity and specificity, but are more intuitively useful in the way that patients present.

The formula for positive predictive value is:

$$PPV = \frac{\text{True positives}}{\text{All positives (true and false)}}$$

The formula for negative predictive value is:

$$NPV = \frac{\text{True negatives}}{\text{All negatives (true and false)}}$$

The same 2×2 table can be used to classify those with Disease and those who are Normal, and those who test + and −. Notice that the denominators consist of the rows instead of the columns.

		Disease	Normal	
Test	+	TP	FP	Total +
Result	−	FN	TN	Total −

Tests with high sensitivity will have few false negatives and therefore a better negative predictive value, whereas those with high specificity will have better positive predictive value. An interesting feature of predictive values is that they depend not only on the accuracy of the test, but also on the prevalence of the disease in the population being tested. This has an impact on whether or not a positive test result is believable.

Even for a test with a high specificity, if the disease is not very prevalent a positive test result will still have a relatively high probability of being a false positive. The following table shows how positive predictive value is dampened by the low prevalence of a disease of 1%, even for a test with high sensitivity and specificity of 99%.[6]

		Disease state	
		D (100 pts)	N (10,000 pts)
Test result	+	99	100
	−	$\dfrac{1}{100}$	$\dfrac{9,900}{10,000}$

$$\text{Positive predictive value} = \frac{99}{100+99} = 50\%$$

The *likelihood ratio* (LR) is a more robust assessment of the accuracy of a diagnostic test. It combines the relatively stable test characteristics of sensitivity and specificity with the clinical usefulness of predictive values. This allows us to account for the *predictive increment* that would be gained by using a test in a particular population.[7] An LR is defined as the likelihood that a particular test result (either positive or negative) would occur in a patient with the disease (D), compared to the likelihood that the same result would occur in someone who is normal (N).

$$\text{Likelihood ratio} = \frac{\text{Probability of test result in patient with D}}{\text{Probability of same finding in patient with N}}$$

Likelihood ratios range from 0 to infinity. The bigger the positive LR, the stronger the argument that D is truly present. As the negative LR approaches 0, the stronger the argument that N is the case. When LR = 1, the test has no diagnostic value.[8]

BAYESIAN LOGIC

The prevalence of a disease is also known as the *pretest probability of disease*. This is akin to asking "In a certain population of individuals with the same symptoms, if we were to pick one at random, what is the probability that they have D?" Bayesian analysis is a tool we can use to improve our diagnostic skills. Bayes's Theorem incorporates the knowledge gained from the results of a diagnostic test that allows us to calculate the posttest probability of the condition using the LR.

A simplified version of the Bayes Theorem is:

$$\text{Pretest Odds} \times \text{LR} = \text{Posttest Odds}$$

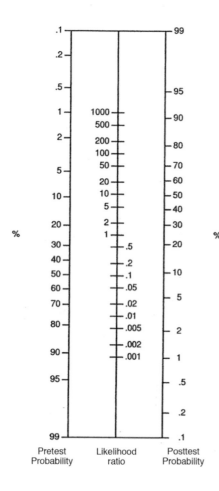

FIGURE 21-3 Nomogram for converting pretest probability to posttest probability, after a diagnostic test with a given likelihood ratio. The odds have been changed into probability in the nomogram. *(From Fagan, T. J. 1975. Nomogram for Bayes theorem. Letter: New Engl J Med, 293:5, 257 with permission.)*

The nomogram in Figure 21-3 has been developed to portray the overall usefulness of a diagnostic test in settings with different pretest probabilities (or prevalence) of disease. The posttest probability reflects the additional knowledge gained by doing the test. Notice that for any line intersecting an LR of 1, the pretest and posttest probabilities do not change. The more extreme LRs have a larger impact on the difference between pre- and posttest probabilities.

In general, diagnostic tests provide the most additional information when they are performed on individuals who have an intermediate probability of disease, somewhere around 20% to 80%. Figure 21-4 illustrates the additional incremental information gained by doing a thallium imaging test (sensitivity of 75% and specificity of 90% compared to the Reference Standard of cardiac angiogram) in diagnosing coronary artery disease (CAD). The largest incremental changes from pre- to posttest probability occur when the prevalence (pretest probability) of the condition is in the moderate range. This holds true for either a + or − test result.

It may be tempting to order a test to confirm or reject a diagnosis, but a test should not be done if the result will not change the recommended pathway. If we know the pretest probability of D or N is very high or low, it is not likely that a diagnostic test will add significantly to our knowledge of the patient's condition. A caveat to this general principle is a condition that could ultimately prove fatal if not diagnosed. In these cases, the threshold for diagnostic tests may be lowered even though they may add only incremental degrees of certainty. One may also proceed directly to the Reference Standard in these cases.

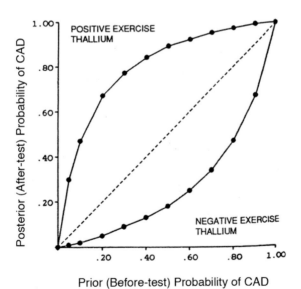

FIGURE 21-4 The posttest probability of coronary artery disease as a function of the pretest probability and the results of a thallium scintiscan. The most knowledge is gained when the pretest probability, which is estimated from the patient's symptoms, is in the moderate range. *(From Goldman, L. 1986. Noninvasive tests for diagnosing the presence and extent of coronary artery disease: Exercise, electrocardiography, thallium, scintigraphy, and radionuclide ventriculography. J Gen Intern Med, 1(4): 258-65.)*

REFERENCES

1. Goldman, L. et al. 1998. *Primary Cardiology*. Philadelphia, PA: WB Saunders Co.
2. Sackett, D. L. et al. 2000. *Evidence-based medicine: How to practice and teach EBM*. New York: Churchill Livingstone.
3. www.blackwellpublishing.com/specialarticles/jcn_11_136, 2006.
4. www.wikipedia.org "receiver operating characteristic", 2006.
5. www.uptodate.com "evaluating diagnostic tests", 2006.
6. Fleming, M. D. et al. 2004. Pulmonary embolism: Diagnostic evaluation. *Amer J Clin Med*, 1:1, 6.
7. Gallagher, E. J. 1998. Clinical utility of likelihood ratios. *Ann Emerg Med*, 31:3, 391.
8. McGee, S. 2002. Simplifying likelihood ratios. *J Gen Intern Med*, 17:8, 646–649.

Afterword

> We didn't inherit the land from our fathers, we are borrowing it from our children.
>
> —Old Amish saying

We have the golden opportunity to bestow many fulfilling life years by applying the knowledge we gain when we use biostatistics to its full effect. Many of us will live our lives to our ultimate lifespan, with most of those years filled with productive and rewarding experiences. This methodology can be used to its full advantage not only through medical treatments, but preventative measures as well.

We have seen amazing advances in the past century. There are many among us who remember the advent of the polio vaccine, antibiotics, and public health laws that ensure safe food and water. Treatments for cancer and end-stage heart failure can extend life longer than ever before. However, not all of the inhabitants of this planet have access to the same health benefits that only some of us enjoy. The challenge of the next century will be to apply the knowledge in ways that bestow QUALYs to people in all parts of the globe.

If we are able to accomplish this ambitious goal, we might be reassured that the best interests of all have been met. However, the power of intervention to improve outcomes can be extended beyond those who are currently living. We can use this knowledge to mold the future so that our descendents will continue to appreciate the benefits that we currently experience.

The population of earth has risen exponentially in the last century to over 6 billion inhabitants, and continues to grow. The consumption of our natural resources is occurring at a continuously faster rate.[1] The result has been a cumulative negative effect on our natural world, and has upset the intricate balance between the environment and the plants and animals that have evolved over hundreds of thousands of years.

This past century has also seen the arms race accelerate to the point where we have created weapons that, when used in the manner that they were designed to be used, are extremely destructive and may even be capable of extinguishing the human race. The damage brought about by political conflicts can undermine the system that provides health and happiness to its people. All the potential QUALYs in the lifespan of an individual, and especially that of an infant, are suddenly devalued in the setting of a war.

173

We have the capacity and the tools to apply our knowledge to the betterment of humankind, not only for limited populations, but for the benefit of the Earth's present and future inhabitants. This is an enormous challenge but one that we must face. The remarkable capacity of humans to solve problems, even if it takes several centuries, is an indication that anything is possible. If we have the ability to achieve our utmost intellectual capacity, we will arrive there when we are able to recognize situations that have detrimental global impact and intervene effectively, while protecting the individual's right to pursue a quality life experience.

Gail F. Dawson

[1]Wilson, E. O. 2002. *The Future of Life*, New York: Random House.

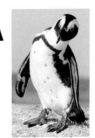

Flowchart of Types of Statistical Tests

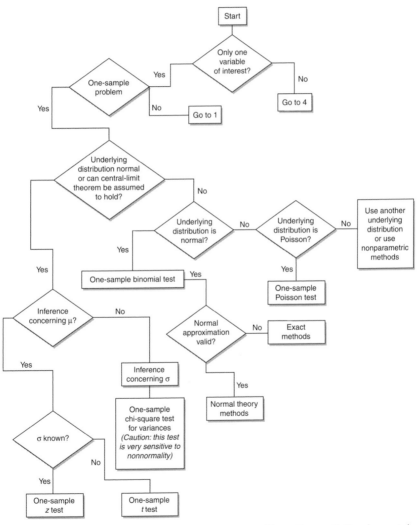

FIGURE APP A-1 Flowchart: Methods of Statistical Inference. *(From Rosner B: Fundamentals of Biostatistics, Duxbury Press, 1999 with permission)* *(Continued)*

175

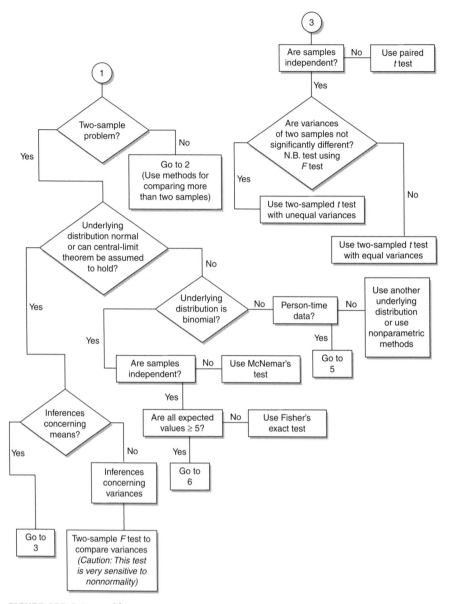

FIGURE APP A-1, cont'd.

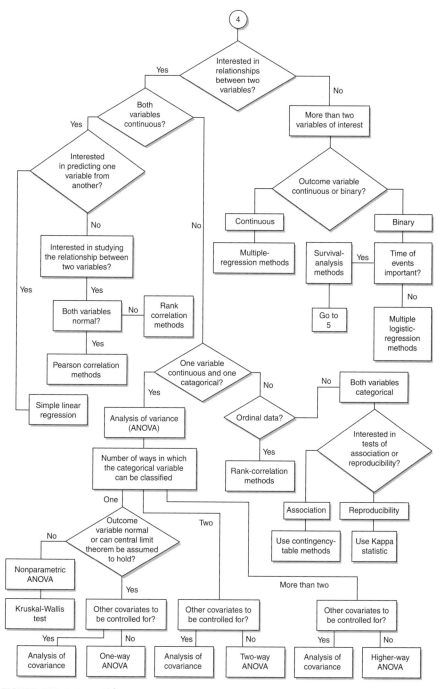

FIGURE APP A-1, cont'd.

(Continued)

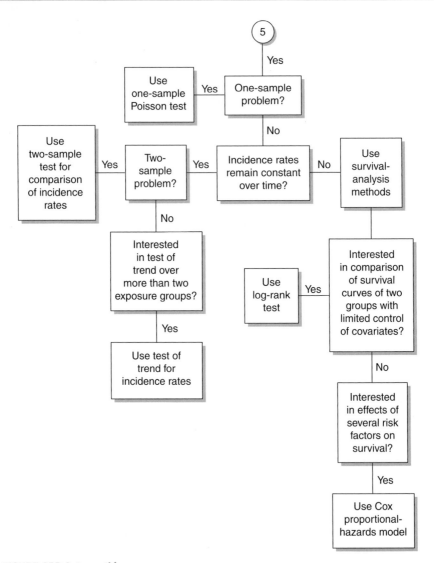

FIGURE APP A-1, cont'd.

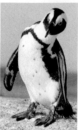

Simplified Flowchart of Types of Statistical Tests

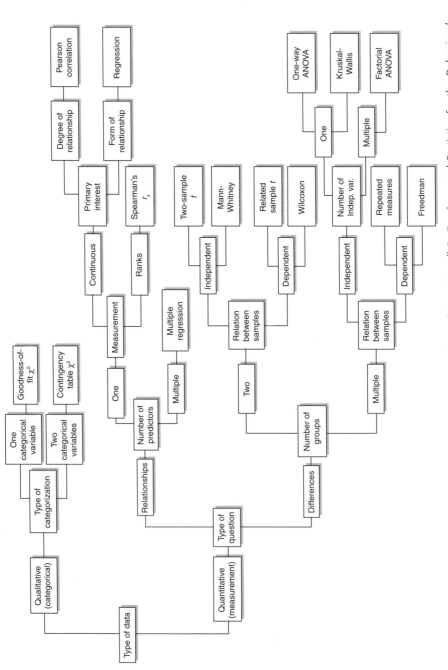

FIGURE APP B-1 A more simplified approach to flowchart in Appendix A. *(From Howell D: Fundamental Statistics for the Behavioral Sciences, 4th ed, Brooks/Cole Publishing Co., Pacific Grove, CA, 1999 with permission)*

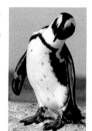

Values of Normal Distribution

Normal Curve Areas

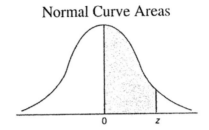

z	.00	.01	.02	.03	.04	.05	.06	.07	.08	.09
0.0	.0000	.0040	.0080	.0120	.0160	.0199	.0239	.0279	.0319	.0359
0.1	.0398	.0438	.0478	.0517	.0557	.0596	.0636	.0675	.0714	.0753
0.2	.0793	.0832	.0871	.0910	.0948	.0987	.1026	.1064	.1103	.1141
0.3	.1179	.1217	.1255	.1293	.1331	.1368	.1406	.1443	.1480	.1517
0.4	.1554	.1591	.1628	.1664	.1700	.1736	.1772	.1808	.1844	.1879
0.5	.1915	.1950	.1985	.2019	.2054	.2088	.2123	.2157	.2190	.2224
0.6	.2257	.2291	.2324	.2357	.2389	.2422	.2454	.2486	.2517	.2549
0.7	.2580	.2611	.2642	.2673	.2704	.2734	.2764	.2794	.2823	.2852
0.8	.2881	.2910	.2939	.2967	.2995	.3023	.3051	.3078	.3106	.3133
0.9	.3159	.3186	.3212	.3238	.3264	.3289	.3315	.3340	.3365	.3389
1.0	.3413	.3438	.3461	.3485	.3508	.3531	.3554	.3577	.3599	.3621
1.1	.3643	.3665	.3686	.3708	.3729	.3749	.3770	.3790	.3810	.3830
1.2	.3849	.3869	.3888	.3907	.3925	.3944	.3962	.3980	.3997	.4015
1.3	.4032	.4049	.4066	.4082	.4099	.4115	.4131	.4147	.4162	.4177
1.4	.4192	.4207	.4222	.4236	.4251	.4265	.4279	.4292	.4306	.4319
1.5	.4332	.4345	.4357	.4370	.4382	.4394	.4406	.4418	.4429	.4441
1.6	.4452	.4463	.4474	.4484	.4495	.4505	.4515	.4525	.4535	.4545
1.7	.4554	.4564	.4573	.4582	.4591	.4599	.4608	.4616	.4625	.4633
1.8	.4641	.4649	.4656	.4664	.4671	.4678	.4686	.4693	.4699	.4706
1.9	.4713	.4719	.4726	.4732	.4738	.4744	.4750	.4756	.4761	.4767
2.0	.4772	.4778	.4783	.4788	.4793	.4798	.4803	.4808	.4812	.4817
2.1	.4821	.4826	.4830	.4834	.4838	.4842	.4846	.4850	.4854	.4857
2.2	.4861	.4864	.4868	.4871	.4875	.4878	.4881	.4884	.4887	.4890
2.3	.4893	.4896	.4898	.4901	.4904	.4906	.4909	.4911	.4913	.4916
2.4	.4918	.4920	.4922	.4925	.4927	.4929	.4931	.4932	.4934	.4936
2.5	.4938	.4940	.4941	.4943	.4945	.4946	.4948	.4949	.4951	.4952
2.6	.4953	.4955	.4956	.4957	.4959	.4960	.4961	.4962	.4963	.4964
2.7	.4965	.4966	.4967	.4968	.4969	.4970	.4971	.4972	.4973	.4974
2.8	.4974	.4975	.4976	.4977	.4977	.4978	.4979	.4979	.4980	.4981
2.9	.4981	.4982	.4982	.4983	.4984	.4984	.4985	.4985	.4986	.4986
3.0	.4987	.4987	.4987	.4988	.4988	.4989	.4989	.4989	.4990	.4990

FIGURE APP C-1 Values of the Normal Distribution. *(From Sternstein M: Barron's EZ 101 Statistics, Barron's Educational Series Inc., Hauppauge, NY, 1994 with permission)*

Index

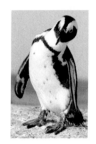